30 STEPS
TO
Finding
Yourself

30 STEPS TO FINDING YOURSELF

Copyright © Sally Hope, 2024

An Hachette UK Company
www.hachette.co.uk

Vie Books, an imprint of Summersdale Publishers Ltd
Part of Octopus Publishing Group Limited
Carmelite House
50 Victoria Embankment
LONDON
EC4Y 0DZ
UK

www.summersdale.com

Printed and bound in China

ISBN: 978-1-83799-145-7

Substantial discounts on bulk quantities of Summersdale books are available to corporations, professional associations and other organizations. For details contact general enquiries: telephone: +44 (0) 1243 771107 or email: enquiries@summersdale.com.

Neither the author nor the publisher can be held responsible for any injury, loss or claim – be it health, financial or otherwise – arising out of the use, or misuse, of the suggestions made herein. This book is not intended as a substitute for the medical advice of a doctor or physician. If you are experiencing problems with your physical or mental health, it is always best to follow the advice of a medical professional.

An Introduction to *30 Steps to Finding Yourself*

Thanks for picking up *30 Steps to Finding Yourself*. This is your opportunity to spend some time with your best friend: you. However, you might not be your own best friend right now: you might currently be your harshest critic. If this is the case, this book should help you to develop a better understanding of the most important person in your life – you! I hope that, on reading these pages, you can start to forge a beautiful, lifelong relationship with yourself.

For many women, there comes a point in their lives when they wonder who they are outside of their relationships. For some, this might happen as early as childhood; for others it may not happen until later in life. But whatever age you are, "Who am I?" is an important question to ask, and the more confidently you are able to answer it, the better your personal growth, happiness, self-esteem and even career success could be.

This 30-step journalling exercise takes you on a unique and personal journey to find your own answers to this question. Each chapter contains five "steps" worth of journals, each building on the last, for you to read and explore. However you choose to engage with this book, I'd encourage you to document your thoughts each day. Don't feel the need to keep this book pristine – write in it, draw in it, doodle, document your thoughts and feelings, and consider this book your travel journal as you embark on this exciting journey. The journalling exercises encourage creativity as a form of expression, but we're all different, so use whichever exercises work for you. It's good to try new things though, so I hope you'll give some of the ones you aren't so comfortable with a try. Pause, reflect and treat yourself with a little loving kindness, and enjoy taking the steps toward uncovering your true, authentic self.

Chapter One

WHAT MAKES ME, ME?

Step 1
Who Cares?

Know thyself.

ANCIENT GREEK APHORISM

"Who cares who I am? I'm just me: I bumble along, taking each day as it comes. I don't need to sit down and think about this stuff, do I?"

Does the above resonate with you? Maybe you've never really given much thought to who you are, what makes you tick, what you love or what really grinds your gears and why. Perhaps you've never really considered what makes you different from other people, what your unique qualities are or what you're particularly passionate about. Do you really need to?

From the time of the ancient Greeks, philosophers, psychologists and wise sages have urged their students on the quest for self-discovery. But why? Why is it important to have a good sense of who you are?

- Having a strong sense of our identity means we can understand our place in the world. If we understand what really matters to us, we can prioritize those things and give ourselves a sense of purpose.

- A good sense of identity boosts self-esteem. How can we learn to love ourselves if we don't even know who we are?

- Strong self-esteem enables us to set boundaries and protect ourselves in relationships. If we understand our own values about what is and isn't acceptable, and we realize we deserve to be treated with respect, we are more likely to be able to build healthy relationships. We've all got one of those friends who gets into a new relationship and begins to change: suddenly they don't like the things they used to like; they don't care about the things that used to matter to them; their values and priorities suddenly change. Perhaps you've been that person? When we don't have a good sense of who we are, it's easy to become "we" in a relationship and lose sight of "me".

- Having a good sense of who we are can help us to be successful: if we know what's important to us, we can focus on it; if we know what our strengths are, we can play to them.

In Chapter Five, we'll be looking at what success looks like for you (it's different for all of us).

Can you think of any other reasons why it's useful to have a strong sense of self?

Imagine the stickwoman below is you. How well do you currently feel you know yourself? A half? A quarter? More? Or less? Colour in the amount of the stickwoman that represents this.

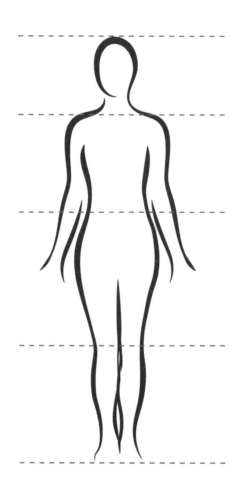

TO THINK ABOUT

Consider why it's important to you to get to know yourself better. Have there been times in your life where you think you might have done something differently if you'd been practising the art of "knowing thyself"? Is there anything you hope for from the future that you think knowing yourself will help with? Think about what you already know about yourself. Do you like it? If not, why not?

TO DO

Over the course of the week, start to make a "Me Collage". Grab a big piece of paper, some felt tips, glue and a pile of magazines. Then find and cut out pictures, or draw and write words that you think reflect who you are and that give a sense of "you". The idea is to think about what makes you unique. It might be a challenge, but do a little bit each day and spend the time considering in more depth who you are. Create something that really celebrates you – the only you there is!

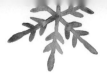

Step 2

What Makes Me, Me?

Today you are you, that's truer than true, there's no one alive who is you-er than you.
DR SEUSS

What's the matter, Snowflake?

In 1885, a scientist called Wilson Bentley attached a microscope to his camera and took some photographs of snowflakes. For the first time, we saw snowflakes in all their intricate detail.[1] We learned that no matter how many billions of snowflakes fall from the sky, no two are ever the same. That's part of their intricate beauty.

The reason why snowflakes are all unique comes down to how they're made: the conditions must be exactly right for snowflakes to form. When it is both cold enough and there is enough water vapour in the air, ice crystals form around tiny flecks of dust or other matter. When it's heavy enough, the snowflake falls from the sky and its shape is formed as it falls through more water vapour.

Even two snowflakes falling side by side will encounter slightly different amounts of water vapour and humidity, so they will form differently. It's the journey the snowflake takes from when it started in the cloud to reaching the ground that shapes it.

We are all like snowflakes: we all start off differently and are formed by the journeys we take.

Do we have a generation of "Snowflakes"? Yes – and you're beautiful. All of you.

---

[1] To see Wilson Bentley's snowflake photographs, visit www.hyperallergic.com/341446/the-first-snowflake-photographs/. To learn how a snowflake is formed, visit www.geology.com/articles/snowflakes/.

Your Snowflake Journey

On the stickwoman below, draw some arrows and write all the things you can think of that have contributed to who you are. You don't need to think quite yet about what your unique features and traits are (we'll get to that in the next chapter), just what has helped to shape them.

For example, if you think that growing up in a large family has helped make you the way you are, you'd write that with an arrow pointing to the stick person.

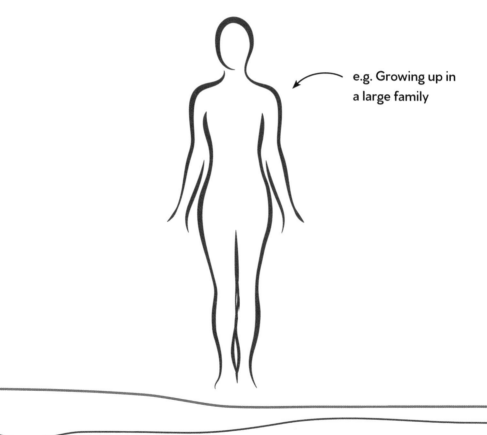

e.g. Growing up in a large family

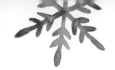

The things you have written around your stickwoman probably fall into three broad categories:

- **Biology/genetics:** These are the things you're born with, for example, your sex, race and innate talents, such as being bad or good at sport or music. Or maybe you have a physical trait that has impacted your life (I know, being 4 foot 10 inches, that I have a touch of "short person syndrome").

- **Experiences:** These are things that have happened to you, such as school experiences, house moves, hardships, successes, failures and so on.

- **Choices:** These are the things you choose to do, such as your job, hobbies and friendships.

Have a look at the things you've written around your stickwoman. Which category does each comment fit into? Are there any that don't fit into these categories? Can you think of any other examples from these categories that may have influenced who you are? If so, add them to your diagram.

Throughout the rest of this chapter, we're going to think about how these things interact with each other to form our individual personality. Then we'll look at each area in turn, starting with our biology.

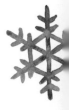

TO THINK ABOUT

What do you think is the biggest factor contributing to who you are? How do you feel about that?

_____

_____

_____

_____

_____

_____

_____

_____

_____

_____

_____

_____

_____

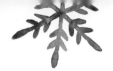

To Do

Make some paper snowflakes! As you spend time cutting them out, consider what your own journey has been. As you unfold them, notice how the beauty becomes clear when you step back from the creative process and examine them. Keep the snowflakes in sight so they can remind you that whatever has shaped you, you have been formed into an intricate, unique, beautiful human.

How to make six-pointed paper snowflakes

1. Begin with a square piece of paper.

2. Fold the square of paper diagonally, to make a triangle.

3. Fold in half again.

4. Fold one-third into the middle.

5. Fold the remaining third into the middle.

6. Cut the point off at the top at an angle.

7. Cut shapes into it along the sides and bottom.

8. Unfold to reveal your unique snowflake!

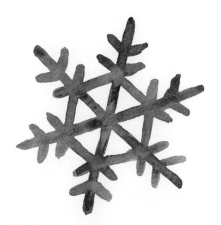

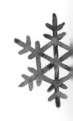

Step 3

My Intricate Journey

> You could not remove a single grain of sand from its place without thereby... changing something throughout all parts of the immeasurable whole.
>
> JOHANN GOTTLIEB FICHTE

The Butterfly Effect[2] refers to the way that even the tiniest, most insignificant moments can make big differences to future events. The notion came from simulating tornados and observing that the flap of a distant butterfly's wings several weeks earlier impacted the tornado. In the same way, seemingly insignificant factors all interact to form the big picture of our personalities. The more we can understand the interaction of these factors, the better we can understand how we tick.

Have a look at the stickwoman you wrote around in the previous exercise. The arrows show that all these factors feed into creating who you are. Now take a pen and add an arrow to the other end of each line to demonstrate that, while all these factors influenced you, you also influenced them. The relationships between who we are, what we experience and what we do work both ways – it's all intrinsically linked.

Our personalities determine the choices we make. For example, an extrovert might go to a party, while an introvert reads a book; a risk taker might climb a mountain while someone who is risk averse chooses a safer activity; some of us revise for the exam, others don't. These choices all determine our experiences, and the experiences shape who we are. Not only that, but our personality also determines how we react to experiences. Some of us are naturally resilient, some of us are optimistic, some of us take risks, while others are better at spotting danger. Again, this affects how our personalities develop. This all suggests that, while we may be born with certain traits, our personalities aren't necessarily fixed. The snowflake that hits the ground isn't the same shape as when it fell from the cloud.

[2] For further information about the Butterfly Effect, please visit: www.americanscientist.org/article/understanding-the-butterfly-effect.

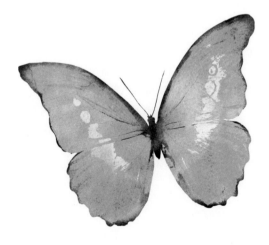

What If...?

This may leave you with a sense of, "What if... ?" We've all played the "What if... ?" game...

- What if I hadn't gone to that party and met the guy I had an awful relationship with?
- What if I'd studied harder and gone to college?
- What if I'd said, "No"?
- What if I'd said, "Yes"?

But regret doesn't get us anywhere; it doesn't change anything. This chapter isn't about "What ifs". It's about:

1. **Considering the relationships between your personality, experiences and choices, and how they have fed into who you have become. In other words, self-awareness.**

2. **Taking control of who you are moving forward.**

Maybe you do wish you'd been more self-confident or more of a risk-taker in a certain situation, or perhaps you can imagine different experiences that would have helped you develop alternative skills or attitudes. Maybe you wish you'd been quieter or more risk averse, or perhaps you can now see how you might have avoided a hardship that's left you with some neuroses you wish you didn't have. While regret is fruitless, learning from your experiences isn't. If you have the self-awareness to understand how your past has shaped you, then you've made the first step in taking control of how you can grow moving forward.

TO THINK ABOUT

Think about the most standout personality trait you have. Write down what you think may have played a part in the growth of this trait – you can probably think of a variety of things that have contributed to it, with one perhaps being, "That's just the way I am". Have any of your other personality traits led to choices and/or experiences that have influenced this one?

TO DO

Remember, guilt and regret are a waste of time. Choose an act of kindness and do it for yourself... it may be running a nice bath, making space to sit down with a book and a cup of tea or simply paying yourself a compliment. Don't skip this activity – find a way to make it your own. It's important to spend time nurturing yourself and treating yourself with compassion and kindness as you discover what makes you tick. Making time for yourself away from the busyness of life will give you an opportunity to reflect on the things you have written above.

Step 4

You Can Be Whoever You Want to Be

> The self is not something one finds;
> it is something one creates.
>
> THOMAS SZASZ

Bonsai trees[3] are grown not by gardeners, but by artists. The cultivator of the bonsai designs the tree in advance. As it grows, they re-pot, prune and graft, to create the tree according to their vision, ensuring the conditions are right for the specific design and removing anything that begins to grow that doesn't visually align.

Contrast this to the snowflake we talked about earlier in the journal. The snowflake, like the bonsai, needs exactly the right conditions to form, but it forms and grows by accident. There is beauty in both, but with the bonsai, the designer decides what that beauty looks like.

Are you a bonsai tree or a snowflake? Is it possible to be like a bonsai tree? Can you be whoever you want to be? If you were like a bonsai tree, have you any idea how you would like to grow?

Neuroscientists now believe that the way our nerves connect in our brain never stops changing and developing. They call it "brain plasticity". The way we live our lives, the things we do and our experiences all physically alter the shape of our brains and, therefore, who we are. As an example, psychologists have found that when taxi drivers in London memorize all the different routes and place names (there hasn't always been satnav!), their brains actually change in shape and size because of this learning.[4]

So, who we are is not set in stone: we can and will change throughout our lives. The question, then, is can we exercise control over how we change, grow and develop?

If we know that our personality is determined by a combination of genetic factors, experience (or environment), choices and actions, then we can work like the bonsai artist to create the right conditions for us to grow in the way we want to.

Sound difficult? It is. It involves challenging your beliefs and doing things that don't necessarily come naturally. It means thinking about where you've been, who you are and what you want to become in the future, and this means understanding your own values and priorities. That's what we'll look at, a little at a time, over the next few chapters. Are you ready? You can do this!

[3] There's an interesting article about bonsai trees as an art form and in philosophical thought here: www.openculture.com/2020/01/the-art-philosophy-of-bonsai.html.

[4] To find out how great London taxi drivers' memories are, visit: www.scientificamerican.com/article/london-taxi-memory.

To Think About

Take a look at the picture of the tree on the following page. On the roots and trunk, write about who you are now and the personality traits you like about yourself that you wish to strengthen. On the branches and the leaves, write about the traits you would like to have. If that's hard, perhaps consider the traits you admire in others to guide you, but remember, you're not trying to be someone else, just more you. Is there anything you think you'd like to prune away?

You may want to come back to this later, as you think about your nature, experiences and decisions.

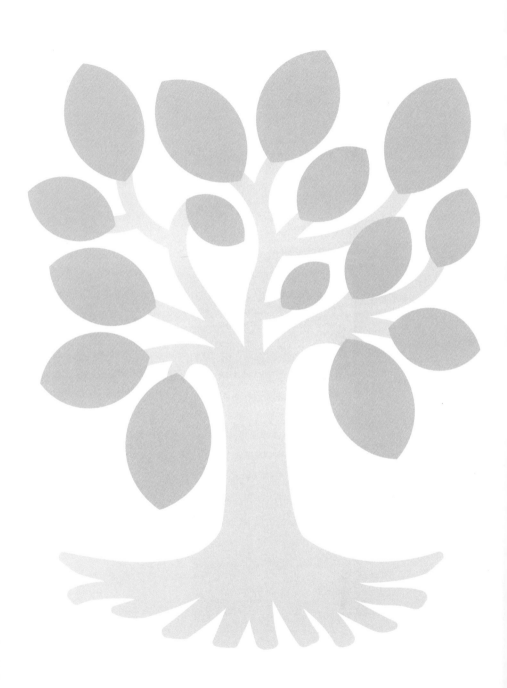

TO DO

To make sure we grow and develop in the ways we want to, we have to be prepared to step outside our comfort zone, to set ourselves challenges and rise to them. This can be scary, but the more often you do it, the less scary it becomes and, before you know it, you're in the habit of doing things you never imagined you'd be able to.

Start practising this with an exercise challenge. Tailor the challenge to your current fitness level, whether it's trying a different training regime or new sport, making sure you have a walk round the park every day or simply increasing your daily step count. Get out there, set yourself a realistic and achievable target and enjoy the pursuit.

Step 5
Labels, Self, Boundaries

> If I am I because I am I, and you are you because you are you, then I am I and you are you. But if I am I because you are you, and you are you because I am I, then I am not I and you are not you.
>
> RABBI MENACHEM MENDEL, THE KOTZKER REBBE

This is one of my favourite quotes, though I must admit that's partly because I like to see the look of confusion on people's faces when I read it out! Think about it for a minute: what do you think it means?

It means that if we base our identities in other people, then we aren't really ourselves. Sometimes, especially if we don't feel confident in our identity, it's easy to base our sense of self on our relationships with others. For example, we may identify as "wife", "girlfriend", "mother" or "daughter".

The problem with basing our identity on our relationships with others is that it's not only bad for our self-esteem, but it means we run the risk of becoming dependent on those relationships. For example, if I identify as "his girlfriend" and the relationship ends, I'm left feeling like I am nobody; I don't know who I am any more. The fear of this may mean I allow him to cross my boundaries and behave in ways that may be unacceptable, because I'm scared that if I challenge him, he will leave.

It's sensible, then, to make sure we're confident and secure in who we are, before forming new, intimate relationships, and it's smart to make sure we don't base our identities in those relationships.

Bake a cake!

If you can, bake (or buy) yourself a yummy cake (if you can't do this, then perhaps imagine a cake). I'd always recommend chocolate, but whatever you choose, make sure it's your favourite. Now, if you can, add some sprinkles to the top of your cake (or imagine them).

What do the sprinkles add to the cake? They're colourful, they look nice and they may be sweet and sugary, and most of us would agree that the sprinkles enhance the cake. But take them away and what's left? A delicious, tasty cake. (You can tuck in now!)

Like sprinkles, a healthy romantic relationship should enhance your life. But if you don't have one, that's fine – sprinkles aren't essential. The cake is still great without decorations, but without a cake, the sprinkles are pretty rubbish. It's important that we concentrate primarily on our cake: ourselves.

Humans are social animals and relationships are important, but no one relationship should completely define who we are.

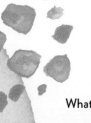

LABELS

It's not just people we might base our identities on. We may give ourselves labels, such as "the mouthy one", "the feisty one" or "the sensible one", or we might identify ourselves by the things we like ("gin o'clock", anyone?).

This is equally unhelpful because we may be tempted to become a pastiche of ourselves – to play to the stereotype and keep ourselves in the box we've put ourselves in. In short, labels limit our freedom.

For example, if you were the girl who always skipped physical education, you may define yourself as "hating sports". This means that when you're grown up, you might miss out on loads of fun stuff, such as canoeing, Zumba or swimming... and all because you didn't like netball or hockey when you were 13!

TO THINK ABOUT

Consider any labels you may have applied to yourself. How do you feel about these labels? Are you ready to let go of them yet? Are any of them positive or helpful?

TO DO

This activity will help you think about the stereotypes you may have applied to yourself, either consciously or subconsciously, and what effects they have had on your life. Take a glass jar with a tealight candle in it. Think about any labels you might have applied to yourself, or any relationships you use to identify yourself. Write these labels on thick paper and stick them to the outside of your jar with PVA glue.

What happens to the light? You can't see it, can you? If we want our own light to shine, we need to remove any labels from our lives.

Now, before the glue dries, take the labels off your jar and replace them with thin tissue paper to make a pretty nightlight (paint over the tissue paper with diluted PVA glue to make it safer and more permanent). Enjoy your candle as a reminder to yourself to let your light shine.

Chapter Two

MY NATURE

Step 6

Who Do You Think You Are?

> Be yourself. Everyone else is already taken.
>
> ANONYMOUS

In this chapter, we're going to take a look at those aspects of your character that come naturally.

In the year 2000, the BBC and The Open University started a project called "A Child of Our Time". Presented by child development expert Professor Robert Winston, they embarked on a project to document the lives of 25 children in the UK born that year, for a 20-year period. The aim of the project was to answer the question: "Are we born or are we made?"

Unsurprisingly the answer was: both.

During the first year of the project, they carried out personality tests on the children. It was fascinating to see their varying responses at less than a year old. For example, to measure levels of resilience in babies, their parents would wear a mask while holding them. We saw how some babies laughed, others looked bemused and some cried: they all responded differently.

If you have children, you probably know that, even from birth, we display different personality traits from one another. In fact, you can probably recognize traits in your children that have always been there. These are our natural traits and they often determine how we respond to situations. It may be that you've grown and changed over the years, but you probably also still have strong preferences toward certain behaviours, even if you sometimes act against that nature.

It's important to recognize our natural tendencies but, as we discussed in the previous chapter, it's also important that we don't define ourselves by them. Developing self-awareness offers us the opportunity to take control of who we become, to develop our strengths, understand our weaknesses, react to conflict and adversity in healthier ways, and more. We will explore this in greater depth in this chapter, but first we need to think about what our natural inclinations are.

Use the sliding scales on the next page to start thinking about what some of your natural personality preferences may be.

What are my personality traits?

On a scale, would I say I am more...

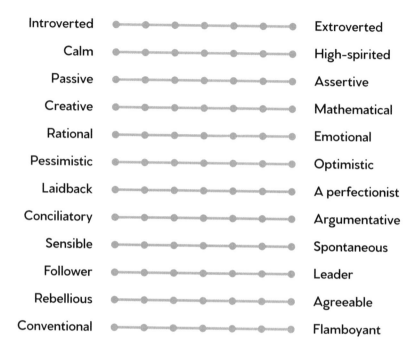

Introverted	Extroverted
Calm	High-spirited
Passive	Assertive
Creative	Mathematical
Rational	Emotional
Pessimistic	Optimistic
Laidback	A perfectionist
Conciliatory	Argumentative
Sensible	Spontaneous
Follower	Leader
Rebellious	Agreeable
Conventional	Flamboyant

Are there any traits you would add to these?

TO THINK ABOUT

Try a mind map. Around the words "I am", write and/or draw all the things that come to mind. Don't think about it too much, just get down everything that comes to mind when you say the words "I am". You can be as creative as you like!

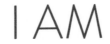

To Do

Celebrate the aspect of yourself you like best! Choose a positive word you feel best sums you up: it can be a word that describes who you are now, or it can be something you want to focus on becoming. Examples might be "caring", "kind", "strong", "passionate" or "determined". Next, find a pebble and write your word on it using paint or a permanent marker (you can add other decorations if you like!). This is your word for the year. Meditate on it, keep it in mind and go back to it whenever you need to. You can keep your pebble in your pocket or your bag as a reminder.

Step 7

OCEAN

> Why fit in when you were born to stand out?
>
> DR SEUSS

How did you find the last step? Was it easy to uncover your natural personality traits? There's a multibillion-pound industry all around self-discovery and personality testing. Psychologists spend years studying what they refer to as "the puzzle of personality", and devising different ways to pin down personality types. Even social media is full of "What kind of... are you?"-type quizzes.

This is because, as humans, we're often fascinated with understanding ourselves, but we find it difficult to do so. If you can't define yourself that easily, don't worry – you don't have to. People are complex, and labels aren't always helpful (as we discovered in the last chapter), so we don't necessarily need to be categorized, boxed and neatly labelled.

That said, considering our nature and personality can be helpful because it can help us understand why we react the way we do in certain situations. It can also help us to work out what we like about ourselves, what our strengths are and where we might need to grow in order to achieve the things in life we want to achieve.

Personality tests can be a useful tool to help us do that, but it's important to remember they're a starting point – a springboard for our own self-discovery. They won't give us all the answers, and they won't give you a hard-and-fast label to pin on yourself – even if they promise that. Lots of people find they get different results on personality tests on different days, as mood can affect how we assess ourselves, so it's always good to remember that these tools are not foolproof. They are, however, a bit of fun and good to provoke thought.

To Do

One of the oldest, most widely accepted and internationally renowned personality models is the Big Five, or OCEAN model.[5] It states that there are five main personality traits. OCEAN is an acronym for the areas of personality it examines: **O**penness, **C**onscientiousness, **E**xtroversion, **A**greeableness and **N**euroticism.

There are lots of online versions of the Big Five test that you can try out for free – a search for "Big Five Personality Test" will provide several options for you to choose from. My favourite has 120 questions and is very thorough. You can find it at www.bigfive-test.com. If you'd prefer something quicker, there's a shorter test available at www.personalitylab.org where there are lots of other personality tests available, too.

Have a go at completing one of these online personality tests and write down your thoughts on the results below.

_____

_____

_____

_____

[5] The Big Five model arose from several independent researchers in psychology and personality. It was initially advanced in 1961 by Ernest Tupes and Raymond Christal, though it didn't rise to prominence until the 1980s. Since then, there has been extensive research, and personality psychologists have reached a consensus that people vary from each other along these five dimensions. Brian R. Little includes a simple version of the test in his book _Who Are You, Really?_ (Simon & Schuster/TED, 15 August 2017; many of the ideas throughout this journal draw on this book and TED talk).

OCEAN
– the Big Five

Here is some information about the five personality areas that the Big Five test measures.

Openness

People who are high in openness are often attracted to new ventures and like to look for different ways to do things. Those low in openness prefer tried-and-tested methods and tradition. They may be more prone to use phrases like, "If it's not broken, why fix it?" Those high in openness to experience are often highly creative and have a tendency to experience emotional reactions to art and music.

Conscientiousness

Those who are highly conscientious are often successful by traditional standards. They generally do better at school and at work than those who are low in conscientiousness. However, these successes are often found in careers and areas where traditional problem-solving methods are encouraged, whereas those high in openness tend to do better at tasks that involve coming up with new ideas and ways of working. Highly conscientious people have good focus and persevere when things are tough; they often have good timekeeping. They are more likely to avoid drugs and dangerous activities, and are more likely to stick to exercise and healthy eating regimes.

Extroversion

Extroverts are reward-driven and crave stimulation. Their need for stimulation and focus on reward rather than punishment means they're more likely to have brushes with authority – be that teachers when they're young or the law when they're older (they get more speeding tickets than introverts). Their musical tastes tend to be loud, pulsing and energizing. Extroverts like social interaction and will often pick quantity over quality in lots of areas of their life.

Agreeableness

Highly agreeable people are peacemakers and will smooth over conflict in a group setting. They also make friends easily. They are often trusting, but might be seen by others as naïve. They are often good at empathy and kindness, and interact with others warmly and expressively. Those scoring low on agreeableness may be cynical and distrustful of others.

Neuroticism

Those high in neuroticism are more prone to depression, anxiety and vulnerability (it doesn't necessarily have to be to clinical levels, though). They are also more likely to experience negative emotions that can interfere with the quality of their life. While an extrovert will seek out potential rewards, someone high in neuroticism is acutely aware of potential punishments and pitfalls. There is a positive side, though: neurotic people are more sensitive. They are astute observers of life, which lends itself well to art and literature, and they spot danger easily. While this may make life harder for them as individuals, society needs their contribution and, from an evolutionary perspective, humanity may not even have survived without them.

TO THINK ABOUT

Consider how your results of the OCEAN test compare with what you wrote about yourself in Step 6. Do you agree with the OCEAN test results? How do they make you feel about yourself?

Step 8

Whose Voice?

> My best friend is the one who brings out the best in me.
>
> HENRY FORD

In the last two steps, I've asked you to consider your personality traits. Now I'd like you to consider – and perhaps write down – how you knew what your personality traits were. What was your evidence? What did you consider to reach the conclusions you did?

It may have been the results of your traits: for example, you may consider yourself "clumsy" because you often drop things or bump into things. Or was it things people have said to you over the years? Things like "You're so generous", or "I really like how compassionate you are"? Or perhaps "You're such a soft touch", or "There you go, picking arguments again"?

I wonder if the things you believe are your strongest personality traits are the things you've heard most? Maybe even since you were a child? Perhaps you hear a voice in your head describing you, saying "You're so...". Whose voice is that? Is it someone whose opinion you respect? It's worth considering how much you value the opinions other people hold about you, and whether they've helped you to form an accurate image of yourself.

Now, have a look at the personality traits you've discovered about yourself over the last two steps. Do you perceive these as positive or negative traits? On the next page, add them to the table.

My positive personality traits	My negative personality traits

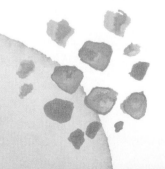

Which traits do you have the most of? If you don't have a fairly even number of both, do you think you have an accurate self-image? Most of us are a mix of both good and bad stuff.

Now have a look again at those negative traits. Are you sure they're all negative? Personality traits are neutral. They're not really positive or negative, they just are – it's what you do with them that makes them positive or negative. For example, some might call climate activist Greta Thunberg "stroppy" or "stubborn", but is she? Or is she passionate and determined to make a difference? David Beckham apparently became such a good footballer because he was always the first to arrive for practice and the last to leave. No doubt many people at the time called him obsessed. He was focused. Many famous artists, writers and scientists, including Roald Dahl, Leonardo da Vinci and Albert Einstein, were called "daydreamers" by their peers, yet they're now recognized as visionaries.

In each of these examples, the person has taken their natural personality trait that could be considered a flaw or weakness and used it as a strength. Sometimes we don't need to work on changing those things we dislike about ourselves; instead we can work on changing how we see them.

To Think About

For each of your "negative" personality traits, consider what it might be called if it were to be viewed more positively.

Here are some examples:

- "I am not bossy, I am a strong leader."

- "I am not a soft touch, I am empathetic."

- "I am not naïve or a pushover, I am warm-hearted and generous."

- "I am not stubborn, I am determined."

Now it's your turn:

I am not _____ , I am _____

I am not _____ , I am _____

I am not _____ , I am _____

I am not _____ , I am _____

Do this for each of your "negative" traits.

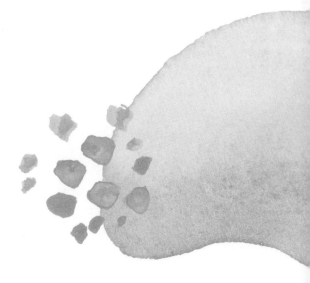

To Do

On the next page, you'll see my "Fuck-It Bucket". The Fuck-It Bucket is a place to chuck all the stuff you don't need in your life any more.

Today we're saying, "Fuck it! I will not be limited by other people's perceptions of me", and *"Fuck it! I will not hide my strengths because other people have told me they are weaknesses."*

So, take those negative words that you've replaced with positive ones about yourself – bossy, stubborn, soft, etc. – and chuck them in the Fuck-It Bucket. You can either write them in the bucket on the next page or, if you're feeling creative, find yourself a bin, bucket or box and make an actual "Fuck-It Bucket" to throw away all the nonsense you don't need in your life any more: write it on a piece of paper and chuck it in.

When you're ready, you can shred the contents of your Fuck-It Bucket, or if you've used the one in here, you can tear out that page and shred it (don't do it just yet though, because I'm sure you'll find more things to put in it before the end of your journey!).[6]

---

[6] This exercise is an adaptation of a popular concept used in a variety of ways. The concept seems to have originated with David Sedaris in his book *Me Talk Pretty One Day*. "When a hurricane damaged my father's house, my brother rushed over with a gas grill, three coolers of beer, and an enormous Fuck-It Bucket – a plastic pail filled with jawbreakers and bite-size candy bars. ('When shit brings you down, just say "fuck it", and eat yourself some motherfucking candy')".

Chuck it in the Fuck-It Bucket

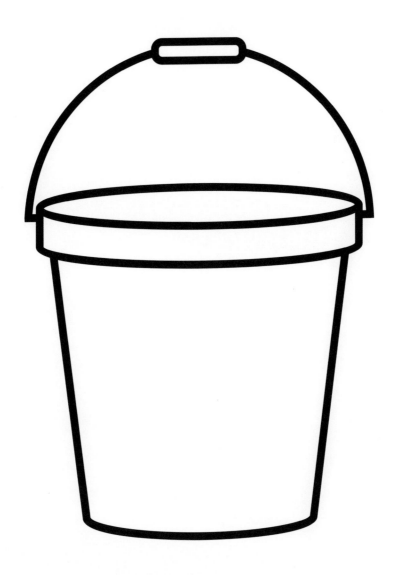

♂

Step 9

Fake It 'Til You Make It

> I pretended to be somebody I wanted to be, and I finally became that person. Or he became me. Or we met at some point.
>
> CARY GRANT

So far, we've considered our natural traits; we've had a think about whether our self-image is accurate; and we've thought about reconsidering how traits we don't like can actually be positive. But what if you don't have a trait that you'd really like to have? What if you want to be something that's contrary to your nature? For example, what if you're a bit blunt and struggle to find the right thing to say, but you find yourself in a tricky legal situation where diplomacy is important? What if you're not particularly conscientious, but you need to study and pass an exam to get your dream job? Or what if you simply really value thoughtfulness, but it's not something that comes naturally to you?

When you did the OCEAN test, did you feel limited by the results? Do you feel limited by having certain personality traits and not others? You don't need to. Scientists have proven that it's possible to physically alter your brain. Wish you were a bit more outgoing? Well, "fake it 'til you make it" and eventually you will be. In other words, imagine what you would do in a particular situation if you were more outgoing, or think of an outgoing person and copy what they do. In other words, pretend to be outgoing. Do this often enough and eventually your brain chemistry will change – you will actually *become* more outgoing. We are not limited by our genetics.

Psychologists also believe that while some of our personality traits are strong, others can be classed as "free traits", meaning they're changeable and adaptable. Jordan Raskopoulos, from the band The Axis of Awesome, describes herself as "shy-loud": she says that while she can play a gig to an auditorium full of people and loves being the centre of attention in other situations, she's socially awkward and very shy. Her introversion is a "free trait", because in some circumstances, she's an extrovert.[7]

This goes some way to explaining why many of us behave differently depending on who we're with. The majority of us don't behave the same way with our closest family as we do with our colleagues, and for some people our personality traits can be flexible. You may have previously thought of this as "being fake", but being able to act in ways that may seem contrary to your nature (when necessary) can be a useful skill to develop. Stepping outside our comfort zones and practising behaviour that's contrary to our natural inclination is how we develop new skills, and it's also a remarkable way to boost our confidence.

[7] You can listen to a brilliant TED talk by Jordan Raskopoulos, where she talks about her high-functioning anxiety disorder, here: www.tedxsydney.com/talk/living-with-high-functioning-anxiety-jordan-raskopoulos.

To Think About

Go back to the "Me Collage" you were working on in Step 1. Is there anything you now want to add to it? Are there any personality traits you don't have just now, but are going to *pretend* you have until you do? If so, add them to your collage.

TO DO

How can you step outside your comfort zone this week? Can you pick up the phone and call to check in on a friend, even though you hate talking on the phone? Or can you perhaps try quietly taking pleasure in spending time alone, even though you're an extrovert who craves the company of others? What can you do? Find one way to challenge yourself to do something differently.

Step 10

Feeding the Monster

> If you hear a voice within you say, "You cannot paint", then by all means paint, and that voice will be silenced.
>
> VINCENT VAN GOGH

When our inner voice tells us who we are, we must consider whether that's an accurate self-image. If that voice is the voice of someone else, we can consider how valuable their opinion is. But what if it's our own voice? Having negative beliefs about ourselves can hinder us from forming a positive self-image, which in turn robs us of contentment, happiness and the confidence to grow.

Imagine our self-belief systems are little monsters who live inside us. The monsters grow depending on how we feed them. What sorts of things do our belief monsters get fed? The food we feed our monster is our thoughts, our feelings, the way we speak to ourselves and our actions. If we think positive, happy thoughts and we do things we are proud of, we'll feel good, as all these things provide our monster with a healthy, nutritious diet, resulting in a happy little monster. In turn, our happy little monster believes we're great and tells us so. We therefore think kindly about ourselves and have the confidence to step outside our comfort zone and challenge ourselves: the whole relationship is cyclical.

However, if we think poorly of ourselves, we feel bad and our actions may reflect that. For example, I may think, "Nobody likes me", which makes me feel sick at the thought of going somewhere new, chatting to another mum in the school playground or joining my friends for a night out, so I don't interact. This affects my relationships negatively and provides my self-belief monster with evidence that nobody likes me. The more this happens, the more likely it is that a passing thought will become a deeply embedded belief that's harder to shift.

What do you feed your monster? Do you find yourself going about your day telling yourself off and believing negative things about yourself, or do you feed your monster a diet of compliments and understanding? Remember, your internal little monster is a part of you. If she's angry or sad, she needs to be treated with compassion and understanding. If a friend was raging at you and calling you names, treating them respectfully as you tried to figure out what had upset them would be more likely to restore your friendship than telling them to get lost, which would likely make them even more upset and angry. When you're mad at yourself, it's the same situation. Giving yourself a pep talk and telling yourself to simply "Shut up" when you're thinking unkind thoughts about yourself won't make the situation better. Rather, your little monster needs to be treated with compassion and kindness; you need to understand and forgive yourself as you start to feed yourself a healthier diet of kindness and affirmation.

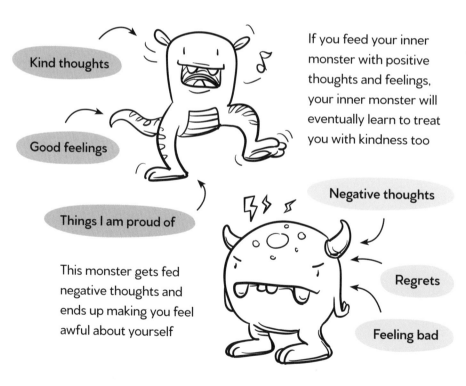

Kind thoughts

Good feelings

Things I am proud of

If you feed your inner monster with positive thoughts and feelings, your inner monster will eventually learn to treat you with kindness too

Negative thoughts

Regrets

Feeling bad

This monster gets fed negative thoughts and ends up making you feel awful about yourself

To Do

Consider your inner monster: what does she look like? If you're a creative type, you might like to make your inner monster: you can draw her, paint her or build her out of LEGO bricks or egg boxes. Whether or not you chose to draw or create your little monster, let's have a think about her diet. You may not have a lot of control over how you feel right now, but you can work on your thoughts. What kind of things are you thinking about yourself that you are feeding to the monster? Write them down here:

_____

_____

_____

_____

_____

_____

_____

_____

_____

_____

If it's negative, perhaps you could chuck it in the Fuck-It Bucket: "Fuck it, I'm not going to think unkind things about myself any more"; or "Fuck it, my inner monster needs a nutritious diet".

Now, we're going to make some good food for our monster. Write down some different things you could think about yourself – positive affirmations (short statements about you that are true, realistic and believable). For example: "I am a caring friend", or "I am intelligent and thoughtful".

Put your favourite affirmation (and your monster, if you made one) where you can see them. Every day, repeat the positive affirmation to yourself, and whenever the negative thoughts creep into your mind this week, challenge them and repeat the affirmation again. Remember, always feed your monster with kindness.

TO THINK ABOUT

Keep repeating your positive affirmation to yourself over the next few days and write about how this feels. Don't expect miracles overnight, though – the bigger and scarier your monster is, the more you'll have to work at those positive thoughts before you see her become a bit sweeter.

Chapter Three

MY EXPERIENCES

You Are a Product of Your Environment

> We are products of our past, but we don't have to be prisoners of it.
>
> **RICK WARREN**

Many psychologists and anthropologists believe who we become is largely determined by our environment – in other words, the situation we live and are raised in. Would you agree?

When you were at school, did you learn the theory of evolution? Charles Darwin figured out that animals had evolved differently around the world by adapting to their natural environment.[8] For example, giraffes have evolved to have long necks so they can eat leaves off taller trees. Indeed, you've probably seen the picture of the evolution of humanity, and can see how humans have become taller and more upright due to changes in our environment and lifestyle. Our environment makes a difference to how we develop physically, but it does so psychologically too.

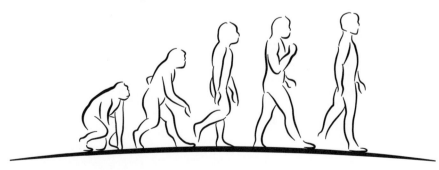

Sometimes, these impacts are obvious: we can look at things we've experienced, particularly trauma, and can point to how they've affected us. For example, if we endured constant criticism as a child, we may feel it has affected our self-esteem. A friend of mine who grew up with seven boisterous older brothers talks about how this caused her to be loud in order to be heard, and thick-skinned from dealing with regular (but loving) teasing.

However, sometimes these effects can be subtle, and we may take on societal beliefs or the expectations of others without realizing we're doing so (in the next step, we'll look at how growing up in a world dominated by men can affect the way we feel about ourselves as women).

A good example of this comes from Nelson Mandela, who grew up and lived under apartheid. How do you think he was affected by racism? The obvious answer is that he was inspired to fight it, and that his experiences contributed to his anger, indignation and passion. But the impact was more complex than that. In his book, *Long Walk to Freedom*, he writes:

> As I was boarding the plane, I saw that the pilot was black. I had never seen a black pilot before, and the instant I did I had to quell my panic. How could a black man fly a plane? But a moment later I caught myself: I had fallen into the apartheid mind-set, thinking Africans were inferior and that flying was a white man's job.[9]

Mandela had, unwittingly, absorbed some of the racist ideology his society had instilled in him, despite spending his life fighting against it.

[8] For further information about Darwin's theory of natural selection, visit: www.bbc.co.uk/bitesize/guides/zt4f8mn/revision/4.

[9] Read more in Nelson Mandela's *Long Walk to Freedom* (Macdonald Purnell, 1994).

To Do

In the picture frame below, consider your experiences. What sort of environment have you lived in? Write or draw all the experiences you can think of that have contributed to who you are. Consider your country, town, religion if you have one (or even if you don't), culture, education, family, friends, the TV you watched and the books you've read. Think of the "big stuff", but see if you can recall any subtle stuff, too. If you want to, or need more space, you can continue this exercise on a separate piece of paper.

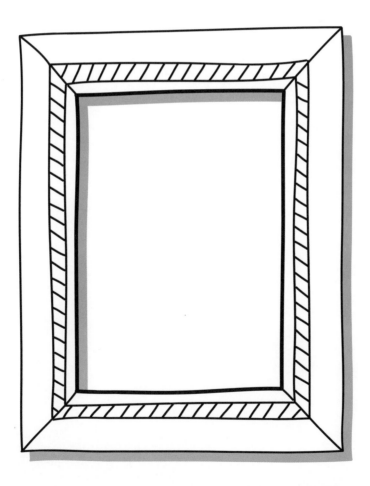

TO THINK ABOUT

Consider the less obvious ways your environment might have shaped who you have become. Can you think of any beliefs you may have subconsciously bought into, like Nelson Mandela did, even though you may not realize it?

Step 12

Twenty-First-Century Woman

> I am a woman with thoughts and questions and shit to say. I say if I'm beautiful. I say if I'm strong. You will not determine my story – I will.
>
> AMY SCHUMER

Are you any good at brain teasers? Have a go at this one:

One day, a man and his son were driving home when they were involved in a horrific car accident. The man was killed instantly, while the son, who needed life-saving surgery, was rushed to hospital. The surgeon raced down to theatre ready to operate, but took one look at the boy and said, "I can't operate on this child – he's my son."

Who was the surgeon? Did you work it out?

Whenever I tell this story in groups, I enjoy watching the leaps we all go through in working out how a boy's dad could have been killed, yet still operate on him: "Was it his stepdad in the car?" "Does he have two dads?" Sometimes someone realizes the surgeon could be his mother, but rarely. I have to confess, the first time I heard this story I didn't get it either.

Despite it being the twenty-first century, we still tend to consider certain traits to be "feminine" and certain traits to be "masculine". This translates into our expectations of the roles men and women will play. On the following page is a list of descriptive words. Grab two different coloured pencils – one to represent masculine traits and the other to represent feminine traits. Without thinking about it too much, circle each word according to whether you feel it's masculine or feminine. Don't match what you think you "should" say – try to go with your gut reaction.

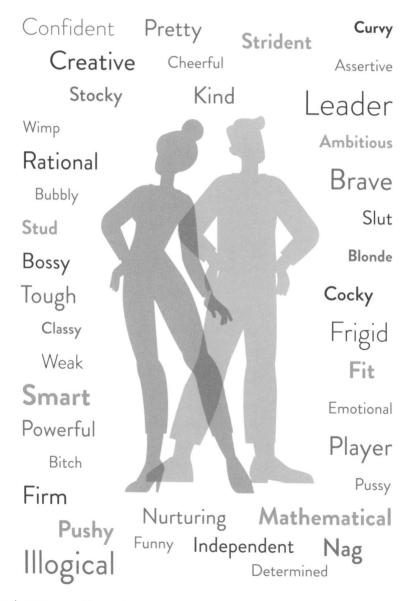

Confident Pretty Strident Curvy

Creative Cheerful Assertive

Stocky Kind Leader

Wimp Ambitious

Rational Brave

Bubbly Slut

Stud Blonde

Bossy Cocky

Tough Frigid

Classy Fit

Weak Emotional

Smart Player

Powerful Pussy

Bitch

Firm Nurturing Mathematical

Pushy Funny Independent Nag

Illogical Determined

When you've done this, have a look at the two groups of words. What patterns do you notice? One thing you may realize is that some of the traits are similar, but they are described in negative terms for men and positive terms for women. For example, you might have decided the word "wimp" is masculine, but the words "nurturing" and "kind" are feminine. This may also have happened the other way around: we may call a man a "player", but a woman "slag"; a man may be "powerful" or "a leader", but a woman is "bossy".

So often, when a man displays character traits we consider "feminine", we describe them in negative terms, and vice versa for women, because – mostly unconsciously – we value different things in women than we do in men. This leads us to have particular expectations of the character traits that people should have and, in turn, the traits that we ourselves should have. This may affect how our character traits develop. For example, if we think of bossiness as a negative character trait, we may withhold our opinions or leadership skills. And if we think of nurturing as a positive character trait, we may work to develop that.

To Do

Have a look at the following character traits and circle the ones you think you have:

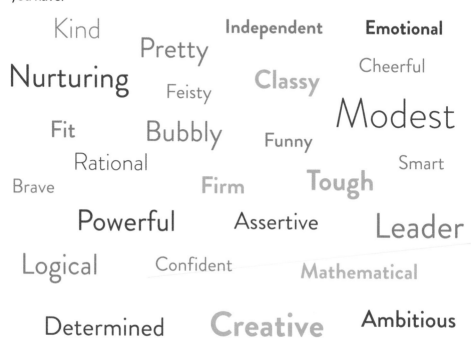

Kind   Independent   **Emotional**

Pretty

Cheerful

Nurturing   Feisty   Classy

Modest

Fit   Bubbly   Funny

Rational   Smart

Brave   Firm   Tough

Powerful   Assertive   Leader

Logical   Confident   Mathematical

Determined   Creative   Ambitious

Add any you think are missing. Despite our unconscious conditioning, ultimately all traits are "human traits", so it's time to celebrate yours!

TO THINK ABOUT

Can you think of a time when you expected something of yourself or someone else based on their gender? Or a time you may have been critical of someone (or yourself) for something you wouldn't have thought twice about had they been a different gender? For example, have you ever referred to a man as being "under the thumb", or a woman as "bossy" or "a slut"? Have you ever chastised yourself for any of these things?

Consider your own childhood. Can you think of any examples where you were given messages about what it means to "be a girl"? Were you ever told to be more "ladylike", or were you treated the same way as boys? Think of the subtle and not so subtle examples.

_____

_____

_____

_____

_____

_____

_____

_____

_____

_____

_____

Step 13

Girl, Woman, Me

> You can't control the cards you're dealt,
> just how you play the hand.
>
> RANDY PAUSCH

In the last step, we looked at some of the expectations society may have of us based on our gender. These notions of which characteristics and behaviours are expected of us are taught to us in a variety of subtle ways by society from childhood.

Did you think of any examples of how you were taught to behave during childhood? Here's a few you might have encountered growing up:

- Giving children toys to play with that are grounded in traditional gender stereotypes. Boys are often given "action toys", such as guns, cars, pirates, soldiers or toys that build engineering skills, such as LEGO blocks, while girls are given toys that encourage creativity, such as art materials, or nurturing/housekeeping, such as dolls and kitchen play sets.

- Responding differently to bad behaviour, using phrases such as "Boys will be boys" to minimize boys' bad behaviour, but telling girls to "be nice".

- Assuming that boys need to run around more, while girls will sit and "play nicely". This can also translate into different teaching styles and expectations in the classroom.

- An unfair division of chores: recent surveys have found that girls still do more chores than boys and that when boys do chores, they earn more pocket money for doing so.[10]

- Traditional fairy tales were usually a story of a girl being rescued by a boy and then getting married. Becoming a princess was her "happy ending". Although films, such as *Frozen*, and feminist rewrites of fairy tales seek to counter this, we still have a wealth of 'tween films, such as *Twilight*, and action films, such as *Jurassic World*, as well as books that follow this stereotypical narrative.

- Media for girls often focuses on appearance. We praise girls for being "pretty", while we celebrate boys for being "tough" or "brave".

Can you add any further examples?

What happens when we don't fit in with these expectations?

What if we're not the sort of girl who cares what she looks like?

What if we aren't interested in having children or we're not maternal?

What if we aren't "graceful" but physically strong, fast or athletic?

What if we're clever but have been told that "Boys don't like girls who are too clever"?

What if we're funny but have been told "Don't be a smart-mouth"?

Even if we do fit in with these expectations, it doesn't mean we don't feel pressured by them. Perhaps we downplay our strengths or try to pretend we have traits we don't. Or perhaps we pride ourselves on being different – on defying societal expectations? Those of us who continue to let our light shine even when it doesn't fit in the "ladylike" box may have been told we're "feisty" or "strident" or "sassy" and, while we may not mind these labels, it's still worth noting that men don't get called "sassy" because they crack jokes or enjoy career success.

In her book, *How To Be a Woman*, Caitlin Moran writes:

> I have a rule of thumb that allows me to judge, when time is pressing and one needs to make a snap judgement, whether or not some sexist bullshit is afoot. Obviously, it's not 100 per cent infallible but by and large it definitely points you in the right direction and it's asking this question: are the men doing it? Are the men worrying about this as well? Is this taking up the men's time? Are the men told not to do this, as it's letting the side down? Are the men having to write bloody books about this exasperating... time-wasting bullshit? Is this making Jeremy Clarkson feel insecure? Almost always the answer is no. The boys are not being told they have to be a certain way; they are just getting on with stuff.[11]

Simply being female in a world that likes to put us into "male" and "female" boxes will have had an impact on the way we have developed.

[10] For more information, visit www.nytimes.com/2018/08/08/upshot/chores-girls-research-social-science.html.

[11] Read Caitlin Moran's *How To Be a Woman* (Ebury Publishing, 2012).

To Do

If you have access to any women's magazines, get your scissors and glue out, and see if you can make a collage of examples of what our culture teaches us to expect of women. Once it's dry, turn it over and, on the other side, have a go at creating a collage of what they teach us to expect of men. If you don't have access to women's magazines, perhaps you can have a look on their websites or Facebook pages to see if you can spot the subtle expectations placed on women there. During the week, look out for examples in the media and everyday life. When we become aware of the subtle messages all around us as women, we can then choose whether or not we want to take them on board.

To Think About

Consider the following questions: Do I feel...

- Pretty enough?
- Free to follow all my interests?
- Free to express my anger?
- Free to share my opinions?
- Able to follow my dreams?
- Clever enough?
- Funny enough?

- Do I need to control/hide my intelligence, humour or talents around men?
- Do I try to be "ladylike"?
- Can I achieve anything I want to in the future? What might stop me?
- Can I behave in the same way as men?
- Why or why not?

Step 14

More Than a Woman

> I can't go back to yesterday because I was
> a different person then.
>
> LEWIS CARROLL

We've considered how gender may have had an impact on who we have become. It's one of the reasons, as we discovered at the start of this journey, that labels might not be useful; if we label ourselves "woman" (or "mother", "sister", "wife", etc.), we may then feel compelled to either rebel against or conform to the expectations attached to that label by our culture.

But we don't only attach labels to ourselves based on our gender. Look back to Step 5. What other labels did you consider that you may have attached to yourself? What expectations does society have of people with that label? How has that affected you?

For example, I am short. There is a stereotype of "the feisty, short one". You may have seen memes about how the short girl in the group is always the loudest or the bolshy one – the one who is "like a Jack Russell". I can see how I've played into and been shaped by that stereotype. I can also identify how other people's expectations of me may have been shaped by that stereotype.

Can you think of anything similar about yourself? If we look at all our experiences in the same detail as we have considered our experience of being female, we can begin to see how we have been shaped in a variety of complex ways that may all interact with each other to create a totally unique experience.

Consider each of these areas of your life (and see if you can think of any others):

- Your nationality
- The area where you grew up
- Your family background
- Your class/cultural background
- Your religion or spirituality
- Your sexuality
- The school you attended

For each, consider whether these "labels" have caused you (or others) to have expectations of who you might be. One way to do this might be to create a mind map. For each, write a word in the middle of the page – for example, you might take "British", "working class", "Mancunian", "Muslim", "single parent" or "survivor" – and write around it all the words that spring to mind when you consider this part of your identity.

Now consider how these expectations have shaped you. Do they match up with who you are? If not, how does this make you feel about yourself? Remember, just because we identify as a particular thing, it doesn't mean we have to meet the stereotype associated with it. People are complex: being a woman doesn't have to mean being graceful and maternal; being short doesn't have to mean being loud and bolshy; being English doesn't have to mean being reserved, and so on. But these expectations can impact us. How have these expectations impacted you? Have they empowered or disempowered you? Have they made you feel good or bad about who you are?

Beliefs

Our experiences can also affect our beliefs. If we have only ever experienced bad romantic relationships, we might now believe that "All men are bastards", or "I am unlovable". It's good to challenge our beliefs, and to ask ourselves how these beliefs have impacted on our feelings and choices.

To Think About

Imagine yourself at an airport with a trolley full of luggage. In your luggage is the sum total of your experiences: your baggage. It's the stuff you're carrying around that other people, society and your experiences (both good and bad) have caused you to carry. You might like some of it and want to hang on to it: perhaps you have some skills or great attributes that you value. Other things, however, might be weighing you down.

Is there any guilt or shame in that baggage?

Are there any feelings of not being good enough?

Are there any feelings of striving to be someone you aren't?

Write on the baggage below what you're carrying around and then decide what you want to keep. If there's anything you want to get rid of, it's time to chuck it in the Fuck-It Bucket – "Fuck it, I decide who I am – not my past."

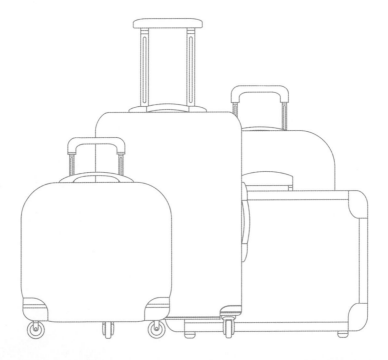

To Do

Since we've been thinking about our childhood, do something today to help you rediscover your inner child. You could do something you loved to do as a child, such as roller skating, climbing trees, playing with toys or colouring. Or pick something you never did as a child: perhaps you never had the confidence to paint or draw, or never jumped in muddy puddles, or built a snowman or had a water fight. Go on – let your hair down and have some fun. Playing is good for adults, too.

Step 15

Better, Not Bitter

> My past has not defined me, destroyed me, deterred me, or defeated me; it has only strengthened me.
> STEVE MARABOLI

The things we experience shape who we are, both positively and negatively. If we can understand how our experiences have shaped us, we can take control of that. We can't choose what we've experienced, but we can choose who we become as a result.

Are there any feelings you've chucked in the Fuck-It Bucket? Maybe you've been left with a sense of shame because of stigma around something you've experienced – well, fuck it! You have no reason to feel ashamed! Or maybe you feel "unworthy" because you don't fit a stereotype. Well, fuck it! Society doesn't dictate your worth! Maybe you feel guilty because you responded to an experience in a way you aren't proud of. Well, fuck it! That's in the past! Guilt is a waste of time.

Are there things you've gained from your experiences that you are proud of? Being small may have meant I've played into the "bolshy" stereotype, but it has also meant I've become determined. I like that. It may have meant I don't always get taken seriously, but it's also meant I've grown a wicked sense of humour. I like that, too. What have you gained from your past experiences that you like?

We'll consider this in more detail later, but for now, a story...

Sometime in the fourteenth century, the shogun of Japan accidentally broke his favourite tea bowl. (I know how he feels – my favourite teacup is currently sitting in my kitchen in two pieces and I'm devastated!) *Distraught, the shogun sent his tea bowl to be repaired, but when it was returned joined together with ugly metal pieces, he was furious. He charged his best craftsmen with finding a more beautiful way to repair his bowl, and thus the art of kintsugi was born.*

Kintsugi literally translates as "golden joinery". It's the art of repairing broken pottery. The pieces are carefully collected and joined with a paste containing gold. The artist does not attempt to hide the damage: rather, it becomes part of the beauty of the object. The pottery becomes both stronger and more beautiful because it was broken.[12]

The story reminds me of my NatWest piggy. In the 1980s, the UK bank NatWest gave away piggy banks to children to encourage them to save. One day, I knocked my piggy off the shelf. It smashed! Like a kintsugi artist, my

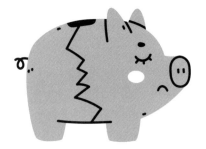

dad carefully collected all the pieces and painstakingly glued them back together. Unlike the kintsugi artist, though, he didn't use gold. He used superglue, and he tried his best to hide the brokenness. I've still got that piggy bank: it sits on a shelf in my bedroom, always positioned to hide its brokenness.

Most of us are a bit broken in one way or another – everyone experiences things that can have a lasting, and negative, impact. What will you do with your brokenness? Will you leave it on the floor in pieces and always grieve for what you think it should have been? Will you repair it with something ugly and spend time trying to hide the brokenness? Or will you repair it with gold and become something stronger, more beautiful and better than before?

[12] To learn more about the art of kintsugi, visit: www.theschooloflife.com/thebookoflife/kintsugi.

TO DO

My favourite teacup is still sitting on my kitchen counter, broken. I'm keeping it, though, because I'm going to plant some tiny succulents in it and make a fairy garden. My hope is that plants will grow through the cracks. Like me, you may not have any liquid gold lying around to make some beautiful kintsugi repairs. But how might you repair something in a way that makes it even more beautiful than before? Have you, too, got a broken pot or cup that you can grow something beautiful in? Do you have a hole in an item of clothing that you can repair in some brightly coloured thread, to add to its uniqueness? It's time to celebrate brokenness.

To Think About

The danger of having unpleasant experiences is that they can make us become bitter, like the ugly metal staples on the first attempt to mend the tea bowl, or the lines of superglue on my poor little piggy. Are there any beliefs you may have developed that you need to challenge to become "better" rather than "bitter"?

Chapter Four

STRENGTHS AND WEAKNESSES

Step 16

Growing Through Adversity

> There is nothing stronger than a broken woman who has rebuilt herself.
>
> HANNAH GADSBY

Life is tough. It's unlikely you've got to the age you are today without facing some challenging times. When we are going through something difficult, we find varying ways to cope.

Imagine living on a desert island[13] where one person has control over everything. What aspects of your life will that person control? Food rations? How your time is spent? Where you live? What else? Write them on the picture on the next page.

Now imagine all the different reactions that might happen on that island and all the different ways those who live there may cope with having so little control. Write them on there, too (you can draw them if you prefer).

[13] This metaphor is based on an exercise from *The Recovery Toolkit*, Sue Penna's 12-week programme for survivors of domestic abuse. There is an accompanying book available: *The Recovery Toolkit* by Sue Penna (Penna & Passmore Ltd, 4 May 2020).

Some people may try to escape; some people might put their head down and comply; others may use violence to rebel; others may collude with the leader and become their friend. When we face adversity, we often feel like we are not in control of our own lives, and there are a number of ways each unique individual may cope with this.

Now imagine a ship sees your SOS signal and rescues you from the desert island. Everyone is returned to their homes and regains their personal freedom. For some people, those coping mechanisms have become a habit and will continue. Some habits that served them well during a crisis may now be unhelpful. However, many of those coping mechanisms could be turned into a skill or strength: those who put their head down and battled on through will have developed resilience; those who colluded with the island's leader may have developed great diplomacy skills. Have a look at the reactions you've written on your island and see if you can think of how they could become a strength.

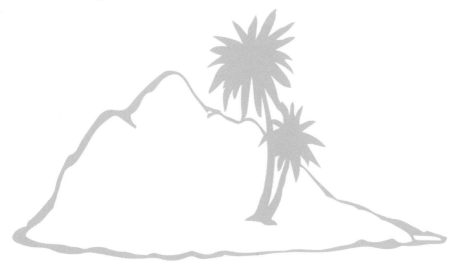

Now, do the same exercise with yourself. Think about the difficult things you have experienced and how you coped.

Some coping mechanisms are:

- Emotional numbing: when we shut off our emotions or build a big emotional brick wall to protect ourselves.

- Fantasy: where we retreat into our imagination, perhaps imagining a better future or pretending that things are okay.

- Covering up: where we pretend to others that everything is all right.

- Collusion: when we collude with a person hurting us, or make a bad situation worse by sabotaging ourselves.

- Anger: lashing out by becoming angry and defiant.

- Compliance: getting on with it, doing as we're told, giving in to a situation or avoiding conflict.

- Avoidance: shifting our focus to food, alcohol, drugs or anything else addictive.

What coping mechanisms have you employed?

TO THINK ABOUT

Write down the coping mechanisms you've used at various points in your life to handle tough times.

_____

_____

_____

_____

_____

_____

_____

_____

_____

_____

Now look at each of these coping mechanisms and think about what strengths they have equipped you with. How can you use what you have learned and the skills you have acquired as a strength? What are you especially proud of about who you have become?

There may be things you're not so keen on, but for now, focus on what is good, better, stronger and more beautiful about yourself. In this step, celebrate that strength. Be kind to yourself: if you've been through some tough stuff and made it out the other side – even if you feel a bit broken and damaged – then you've done something amazing. You are amazing.

To Do

Find a way to remind yourself of your strength every day. Here are some ideas you could try:

- Create a positive affirmation to say to yourself in the mirror: "I am..."

- Write yourself a letter of encouragement as though you're your own best friend.

- Make yourself a "Well done" card.

- Create some artwork around the word that best describes your strength.

- Do something that uses your strength.

- Share your strengths with someone else – be openly proud of yourself.

Step 17

A Bit of Rewiring

Your brain is the most adaptable, modifiable organ in your body, and it can change both positively and negatively by how you use it each day.

SANDRA BOND CHAPMAN

The saying goes, "That which does not kill you makes you stronger". This was our focus in the last step. However, this adage is not always true. Sometimes tough times don't make us feel stronger: sometimes we develop coping mechanisms that become habits that we don't feel able to turn into a positive. Sometimes we develop thoughts, feelings and behaviours we don't like.

This is because we learn by forming connections between events, thoughts and feelings, so eventually our reactions become automatic. This starts in infancy but continues throughout our lives. Maybe, as babies, we smile and someone smiles back at us. This feels nice, so we form a connection between smiling and feeling good. But perhaps we cry and, instead of being fed, we are shouted at. Our brain then forms a connection between crying, shouting and fear, so we learn to be quiet. As our life progresses, this "brain wiring" continues, affecting how our bodies respond to external stimuli. Our coping mechanisms, therefore, can become a hard-wired response.

An example: When I first stopped living with my abusive husband, I found myself feeling fearful and anxious for no reason at 9 p.m. every night. Eventually, I worked out that this was the time he used to come home from work; that in my previous life, 9 p.m. was the time I would be on pins, fearfully getting everything ready for his return. Even though I was now safe, I was feeling anxious because my brain had formed a connection between being unsafe and 9 p.m.

Do you have any thoughts, feelings or coping mechanisms like this? Using a **pencil**, draw or write on the picture of the brain any unhealthy connections you may have formed.

The amazing thing about brains is that they are constantly being rewired – and we can make this happen intentionally. We do not have to be products of our past. Our brains can physically be changed, rewired and rewritten – it's a scientific fact.

Why are pencils made with little rubbers on the end of them? Because people make mistakes. And that's okay.[14] We can take a rubber and erase the bad wiring in our brains. Of course, we can't erase our past, but we can replace the lessons we've been taught if we don't find them useful. Go on, do it now: take a rubber and erase those things you've written on your brain on the opposite page.

Of course, it's not that easy in real life. But it is possible. It takes hard work and practice, but if every time we find our thoughts or feelings defaulting to the negative, if we feel like responding in ways we know are not helpful, then we remind ourselves of the better option.

For example: When I realized I was feeling unsafe at 9 p.m. every night, I started by reminding myself that, in fact, I was safe. I reminded myself of the steps I'd taken to ensure my safety. I then started closing my curtains and making sure my environment was calm and different from how it used to be. I started to distract myself from unnecessary anxiety with a relaxing or fun activity that lasted for an hour, beginning at around 8.30 p.m. I don't even notice 9 p.m. come and go any more.

[14] I heard this observation on Phoebe Waller-Bridge's stage play *Fleabag*, which is also an excellent series available on BBC iPlayer and other streaming services.

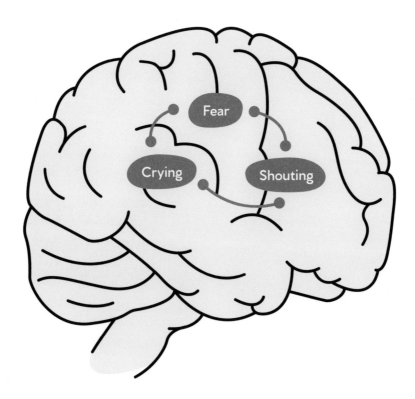

TO THINK ABOUT

What steps can you take to start rewiring your brain to respond differently when you need it to? For example, if something is triggering you to panic, you could start thinking about what makes you feel calm. Or if there are things that make you feel sad or depressed, what can you do in those times to feel uplifted? Or you might wish to use a personal mantra, to regularly remind yourself of the lesson you need your brain to learn – for example, "I am safe, I am loved".

To Do

As we have been considering our weaknesses in this step, it's important to move our focus away from the negative. Start by writing down what you want to get rid of and chucking it in the Fuck-It Bucket.

Now, we're going to try a simple breathing exercise to promote a calm, positive mindset:

1. Find a comfortable position to sit in, with your hands resting gently on your knees.

2. Close your eyes, straighten your back and focus on relaxing your body.

3. Take a deep breath in through your nose, fill up your chest and tummy, trying to inhale slowly for a count of 7 seconds.

4. As you inhale, picture yourself breathing in goodness, warmth, love, strength, power.

5. Hold on to that breath, allowing your body to absorb all the goodness.

6. Now, breathe out as slowly as you can through your mouth, aiming for 7 seconds or more. As you exhale, picture any negativity or bad thoughts you may be thinking about yourself leaving your body.

7. Repeat three times, or more if you prefer.

Inhale the good shit. Exhale the bullshit – you don't need it any more.

Step 18

I'm Okay

> I realized that I don't have to be perfect. All I have to do is show up and enjoy the messy, imperfect and beautiful journey of my life.
> KERRY WASHINGTON

Take a minute to think about someone you know well and love. I imagine you could tell me their flaws. Think for a minute about those things.

Perhaps when you think of the flaws of the person you love, you smile. My sister and I joke about our dad's inability to look at anything in a shop without touching it. We fondly laugh that our dad is like a mischievous five-year-old. Even his more difficult flaws make him who he is. He'd be boring without them. Do you feel the same about the person you've chosen?

Now, think about your own flaws. Do you feel the same affection for them? Or were you less gentle about your own weaknesses? I know I sometimes have far less tolerance for my own failings.

It's admirable to choose to grow – to build strengths and minimize weaknesses. But it's also important to be kind to ourselves and to accept that it's okay not to be perfect.

You have the right not to be perfect.

I have a set of coasters made from reclaimed pottery; part of their charm is that the imperfections in the firing process are clearly visible. Though they all bear the same pattern, each coaster is unique because they all took on slightly different imperfections. In the same way, our flaws are part of what makes us individuals.

In the 90s, models were heavily airbrushed on the covers of glossy magazines. Today, social media encourages us to edit and airbrush our entire lives. We share our highlights: we humblebrag and share picture-perfect photos of #blessedfamilytime, while failing to mention the fact we'd taken a hundred photos just to get one where nobody was scowling or picking their nose. All this leads to us comparing our real lives to other people's curated lives, and feeling guilty when we aren't baking our own bread or hitting the gym. Even when we're focusing on feeding positive thoughts to our inner monster, there's the temptation to beat ourselves up when we don't feel positive. And that's all before we even think about the constant pressure to look good.[15]

It's okay not to be okay.

It's important to accept yourself, "warts 'n' all", because perfection is really fucking boring! Who wants to be perfect? Even Mary Poppins was only "practically perfect". When we choose to love our authentic, flawed, beautiful selves, we give other people permission to do the same; we effectively refuse to buy in to the fakery that causes so many of us to feel "less than".

You're okay just the way you are.

It may seem like a contradiction, but it's not: it's balance. We balance encouraging ourselves to think positively with accepting it's okay to feel a bit rubbish sometimes; we balance trying to grow as people with accepting that we're great the way we are; we balance pushing ourselves outside our comfort zone with taking a break and being kind to ourselves.

[15] Gill Sims' *Why Mummy Drinks* (HarperCollins, 2017) is a humorous and light-hearted story that highlights how women often hold themselves to ridiculously high standards and compare their real lives to other people's curated lives. Highly recommended (even if you're not a mum)!

TO THINK ABOUT

Could you be kinder to yourself? Do you speak to yourself the way you would speak to your best friend? Do you ever struggle with the balance between pushing yourself and allowing yourself to rest?

TO DO

Nothing. Take some time to do nothing. Achieve nothing. It's okay to rest. If the weather is nice, why not spend a bit of time just sitting outside, looking at the clouds and listening to the birds singing?

Step 19
Using My Superpowers for Good

> Everybody is a genius, but if you judge a fish by its ability to climb a tree, it will live its whole life believing it is stupid.
>
> ANONYMOUS

Not all our strengths and weaknesses come about because of our experiences. Perhaps you're naturally artistic or creative, or perhaps everyone in your family is good at singing. Take some time to consider one natural strength you have, as well as one natural weakness. Write them here:

As with your character traits (which we explored in Step 8), it's worth asking yourself what the evidence is that these things are your strengths and weaknesses? Is it because of successes and failures you've had? Are you acknowledging a genuine weakness, or do you have feelings of inadequacy because of things other people have said to you, or pressure that has been put on you by others? For example, if you have been pressured to be more "ladylike", you may feel you are clumsy or insensitive, whereas if you were a man, you may never have even noticed these things.

Take another look at your strength and your weakness. What makes the strength "a strength"? What makes the weakness "a weakness"? I have been told I'm blunt, and maybe I am, but there are times when cutting to the chase and saying what you mean can be really helpful. I may never work as a diplomat, but I bet I'd be much more effective in communicating in situations where speed and clarity are important. Maybe I have a tendency to be pessimistic – fair enough – but I'd be really good at spotting potential pitfalls and dangers, and could work well in health and safety.

When we did the OCEAN personality test, we were told what a high score meant in terms of potential successes and failures. For example, we read that people low in conscientiousness may be more likely to break the rules and get in trouble, but we also learned that they're really good at thinking outside of the box and finding new ways to do things.

Our strengths and weaknesses are often the products of character traits: neither positive nor negative in and of themselves, but with the potential to be either. Look at your strength – what could be the downsides of that? And your weakness – how could it be useful? One of my weaknesses is that I get obsessed with things that are important to me and won't shut up about them; my strength is that I'm passionate, determined and get things done – it's the outworking of the same character trait.

Recognizing this means we can focus on channelling our superpowers for good: I know I can fall into the trap of single-minded obsession, so I make sure I build time into my day for a variety of activities, and I check myself when I'm talking to others about my passions to see if their eyes have glazed over! But I also look for opportunities to work on projects that are important to me, because I know I will have success on seeing things through to completion.

TO THINK ABOUT

Consider what your superpower is. Just as the Hulk has to be careful not to crush things, Cyclops has to wear sunglasses so he doesn't kill people with his laser vision and The Flash needs to slow himself down from time to time, what do you need to do to keep your superpower in check? And what opportunities can you find to use your superpower for good?

To Do

Just for fun, draw yourself below as a superhero! Or, if you're feeling super creative, draw yourself in a comic strip to remind yourself of how you can use your superpowers to save your own little corner of the world. And remember, you don't need to save the whole world – just your little bit of it.

Step 20

Growing Stronger

God, grant me the serenity to accept
the things I cannot change, the courage
to change the things I can and the wisdom
to know the difference.

THE SERENITY PRAYER, REINHOLD NIEBUHR

The serenity prayer is often used by people recovering from addiction.[16] It reminds them to focus on what they have control over right now. It's a useful lesson for everybody.

Similarly, in his book, *The Seven Habits of Highly Effective People*,[17] Stephen Covey writes about a circle of concern and, within it, a circle of control. Our circle of concern contains all the things we care about, including things we cannot do anything about. Within that, our circle of control contains the things in our life we have direct control over. What do you have complete control over?

The only thing any of us has complete control over is ourselves: our own thoughts, our own reactions, our own choices.

If we spend time focused on the things within our circle of concern that are outside our control, we will waste our time. If we spend our time focused on our circle of control, we will build our strengths, recover from traumas and achieve personal growth and successes. As a result, we will gain more control over more things, our circle of control will grow and we will be happier.

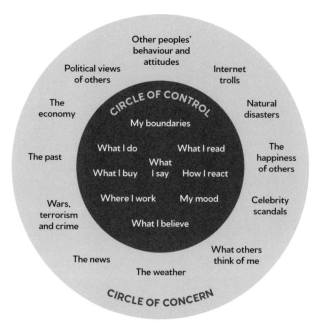

Other peoples' behaviour and attitudes

Political views of others

Internet trolls

The economy

CIRCLE OF CONTROL

My boundaries

Natural disasters

The past

What I do   What I read
What
What I buy   I say   How I react

The happiness of others

Wars, terrorism and crime

Where I work   My mood

What I believe

Celebrity scandals

The news

What others think of me

The weather

CIRCLE OF CONCERN

For example, I may feel that a policy implemented by my superiors at work is wrong. If I spend my time complaining about it, rather than focusing on my own job, then I'm likely to get a reputation as a negative employee. I may even neglect my own duties and end up being reprimanded. However, if I focus on myself, building my own strengths and working diligently at my job, I'm more likely to be promoted, which will put me in a position to influence company policies – thus, my circle of control has grown.

When considering our strengths and weaknesses, it's useful to focus on the things we have direct control over. We will be more successful at building our strengths than if we're worrying about things we can't do anything about. It's also useful for managing anxiety, because we can let go of these things instead of worrying about them. It's time to focus on what we can do.

[16] You can read a little information on the serenity prayer and its use in 12-step programmes here: www.verywellmind.com/the-serenity-prayer-62614.

[17] Read more in Stephen Covey's *The Seven Habits of Highly Effective People* (Free Press, 1989).

To Do

Fill out your own circles of concern and control. What are you going to focus on in your circle of control this week? What are you going to chuck in the Fuck-It Bucket from your circle of concern?

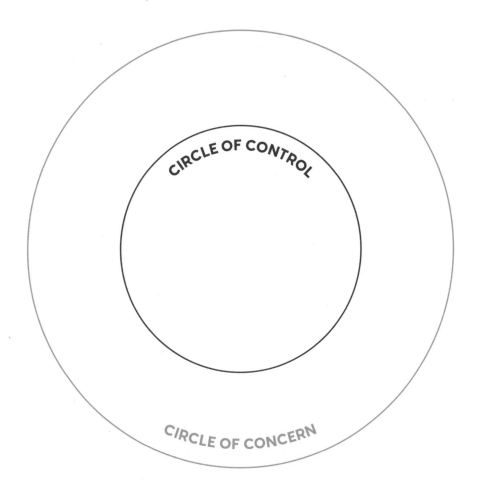

Top Tips

Finally, to finish thinking about strengths and weaknesses, here are my top tips on how to build your strengths...

- Turn your weaknesses into strengths: for example, don't be "stubborn", be "determined"; don't be "interfering", be "caring"; don't be "aggressive", be "passionate". Channel your superpowers for good!

- Practise what you're good at AND what you're not so good at.

- Set yourself goals.

- Step outside your comfort zone – do one thing every day that frightens you, even if this isn't directly related to the thing you want to work on. Getting used to challenging your fears will create good habits for growth.

- Take small steps. Remember, "The journey of a thousand miles starts with a single step" – you don't have to change overnight.

- Take opportunities, join clubs, volunteer and take chances to make new friends: get out there!

- Focus on what you can do, not on what you can't.

And don't forget to be kind to yourself and love yourself in the process. You are already enough!

TO THINK ABOUT

Are there any practical steps you can take from the top tips to build
your strengths?

_____

_____

_____

_____

_____

_____

_____

_____

_____

_____

_____

_____

_____

Chapter Five

YOU ARE WHAT YOU DO – AND MORE

Step 21

You Are What You Do

> We are what we repeatedly do. Excellence, then, is not an act, but a habit.
>
> **WILL DURANT**

Do you agree with this quote? Are we what we do? What does it even mean?

Mostly, we judge others – and are judged – on our actions. This is why people seek to leave legacies behind. In many ways, we are what we do, or at least we are known for what we do.

What we choose to spend our time doing can affect the shape of our brain. We use positive affirmations and challenge our thoughts because this creates new pathways in our brains. We "fake it 'til we make it" and practise new skills until they become habit. What we think and do makes a difference to how we develop neurologically, making us who we are. So, if you want to become a calmer person, you may seek activities that calm you; if you wish you were more of an extrovert, you may plan more social activities. We grow most when we challenge ourselves by doing activities we wouldn't normally do. So, if an opportunity to try something different arises, go for it.

As well as seizing random opportunities, if we're going to take charge of who we are it's a good idea to plan to do things that help us become who we want to be:

I have some sunflower plants on my windowsill. As they have started to grow, they are leaning into the sunlight. I don't want wonky sunflowers. So, every time I water them, I turn them around so they lean a different way every few days. I am controlling the direction my sunflowers grow, just like the bonsai grower pruning her tree. In the same way, we can take action so that we grow in the direction we choose.

But only if we know what that direction is.

To Do

Over the next two steps, we will start to think about what matters to us so we can work out how we want to grow. Before we do, let's establish how we already spend our time. I'd like you to make a "To Do" list. Include every action that's taking up your time, from the mundane, such as "Clean my teeth" to the bigger things such as "Learn to be more assertive". Here's my to-do list for today, as an example:

1. Wake up; turn off alarm.
2. Put the bin out.
3. Wake the children in time for school.
4. Make a cup of tea and a coffee for Mr Sally.
5. Make sure children are getting breakfast.
6. Read social media, check emails, check mobile banking, drink tea and have some quiet time with Mr Sally.
7. Encourage children to put their breakfast pots in the kitchen.
8. Tell children to get dressed and brush teeth.
9. Brush children's hair.
10. Make lunch for Mr Sally.
11. Kiss children, tell them to have a nice day and make sure they're wearing a coat and leaving on time.
12. Kiss Mr Sally and arrange when he will next visit.
13. Doom scroll social media.
14. Make another cup of tea and eat breakfast.
15. Watch TV with breakfast.
16. Clean teeth, shower; get dressed.
17. Put laundry on.
18. Wash pots.
19. Check email and doom scroll social media again.
20. Write.
21. Eat lunch.
22. Read a chapter of current book.
23. Check email and social media again.
24. Collect child from school.
25. Talk to child about their day, tell them well done for anything they're proud of and listen to any problems.
26. Play LEGO with child.
27. Welcome other child home from school, ask them about their day and tell them you are proud of them.
28. Fill out life admin forms.
29. Cook meal planned for today.
30. Listen to children complain about dinner. Encourage them to eat.
31. Watch a TV show with children.
32. Wash pots with children.
33. Put laundry in dryer.
34. Send children to clean teeth and go to bed.
35. Go upstairs and remind children to clean their teeth and go to bed.
36. Make a cup of tea.
37. Go back upstairs and stand over children until they've cleaned their teeth and got into bed.
38. Eat some chocolate.
39. Build a bag of LEGO while listening to a podcast.
40. Take book and glass of water up to bedroom before 11 p.m.
41. Check children are sleeping.
42. Clean teeth.
43. Social media.
44. Read a chapter of book in bed.
45. Go to sleep.

_____'s to do list

_____   _____

_____   _____

_____   _____

_____   _____

_____   _____

_____   _____

_____   _____

_____   _____

_____   _____

_____   _____

_____   _____

_____   _____

_____   _____

_____   _____

TO THINK ABOUT

What thoughts spring to mind when you look over your To Do list? When I've done this exercise in group sessions, many women have remarked, "Woah... I do so much, and so little of it is for myself!" Maybe you feel the same, or maybe you feel your list is a bit short.

Don't beat yourself up – whichever it is, there is value in being busy and there's value in resting. A To Do list can help you to focus on keeping busy, or on simply getting the minimum done when you're feeling overwhelmed. If you're feeling overwhelmed, maybe put some ticks on it when you do those little things, such as having a shower – it can make you feel better.

Step 22

Do What Matters

> Carpe diem. (Seize the day.)
>
> **LATIN MOTTO**

If we're going to make sure we do the things that will help us to become the person we want to be, then we need to know who that person is. To understand what we want to become, we have to identify what is important to us.

We all have different values and we all prioritize our values differently. To identify which personal values are important to you, it sometimes helps to look at what you value in others. Who are your role models? What, in particular, do you admire about them? Are these the values you would like to hold? Or think about what you value in a friendship: what are the deal breakers in a friendship? What makes you warm to a person? This can give you an idea of what you value.

When we act in ways that go against our values, it's uncomfortable: it jars with our sense of well-being. Even if what we're doing is something well meaning, such as telling a friend a lie to spare their feelings, for someone who deeply values honesty, this can cause discomfort. So, it's good for our self-esteem and general feeling of wellness if the things we do can match up to what really matters to us. When we do the things we value, we feel good about ourselves.

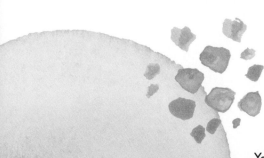

To help you work out what your values are, have a look at the list of words below and highlight the ones most important to you:

Accountability	Determination	Love
Accuracy	Diligence	Loyalty
Achievement	Discipline	Making a difference
Adventurousness	Diversity	Obedience
Ambition	Empathy	Openness
Assertiveness	Enjoyment	Order
Balance	Enthusiasm	Originality
Being the best	Excitement	Positivity
Belonging	Expertise	Practicality
Boldness	Fairness	Preparedness
Calmness	Faith	Professionalism
Carefulness	Family	Reliability
Challenge	Fidelity	Resourcefulness
Cheerfulness	Fitness	Restraint
Clear-mindedness	Focus	Self-control
Commitment	Freedom	Selflessness
Community	Fun	Self-reliance
Compassion	Generosity	Sensitivity
Competitiveness	Growth	Spontaneity
Consistency	Happiness	Stability
Contentment	Hard work	Strength
Continuous	Health	Thankfulness
improvement	Helping society	Thoroughness
Contribution	Holiness	Thoughtfulness
Cooperation	Honesty	Timeliness
Correctness	Humility	Tolerance
Courtesy	Independence	Traditionalism
Creativity	Inquisitiveness	Trustworthiness
Curiosity	Insightfulness	Understanding
Decisiveness	Intelligence	Uniqueness
Dependability	Justice	Usefulness

If there are any other values that are important to you that are not included in this list, add them here.

_____

_____

_____

_____

When you have worked out your personal values, it's also a good idea to work out what your priorities are. What do you really care about? What makes you excited, angry, passionate? This way, you can work out what your goals should be.

You may already have a clear idea of what's important to you. I know someone who is absolutely driven and passionate about making life better for disabled people: she is chair of a disability charity. I know someone else who says he doesn't care about career or money or changing the world: he just wants to be able to spend his weekends on the top of a mountain, because mountain air makes him feel alive! Both are valid. Some of us are spurred on by anger at injustice, others by love, some by ambition and others still just want a quiet life. What are your priorities?

If you aren't sure, have a look at the words below. Do any of them make you feel something? Anger? Determination? A sense of joy?

Healthcare	Homelessness	Books
The environment	Addiction	Sports
Animals	Sexuality	Nature
Schools	Poverty	Outdoors
Benefits	Politics	Family
Children	Fairness	Relationships
Religion	Me	Friendship
Spirituality	Fun	Human rights
Women	Hobbies	
Sexism	The arts	

TO THINK ABOUT

What are your values – what do you want to be known for?

What are your priorities – what do you want to achieve?

What do you want to achieve over the next week/month?

What do you want to achieve over the next year?

What is your long-term life goal?

It's okay if you don't have the answers to that one yet. You can always focus on the first one. And if the thing you want to achieve is watching every episode of your favourite TV show or building an awesome LEGO castle, then that's okay, too – you're in good company!

_____

_____

_____

_____

_____

_____

_____

_____

To Do

Consider making a "bucket list" – a list of things you want to do before you "kick the bucket"! Make it as long or as short as you like, and don't just include big challenges: think about small, everyday "fun" things you might never have done, such as building a snowman or dancing barefoot in the rain. Make sure your bucket list aligns with your values, includes things you want to achieve that are important to you, encourages you to try something you might find scary and broadens your horizons. Have fun with it!

Is there anything on it you can do this week, or this month? Or something you can start to work toward?

Step 23

Hopes and Dreams

> Live out of your imagination,
> not your history.
> **STEPHEN COVEY**

I love hearing people's dreams: the bigger and wilder the better. Mine, by the way, is to retire and travel round the north coast of Scotland in a camper van full of books and tea.

Sometimes, if we've been through tough times, we may feel we dare not dream. But having a vision for the future is good: it's healthy and it can be something to hold on to when times are difficult. During the COVID-19 lockdown, I spent a lot of time driving that camper van round beautiful Scottish roads – all in my head, of course.

What did you hope for when you were younger? Did it happen? If not, is it still a possibility?

Sometimes unfulfilled dreams can leave us with a sense of regret. If you ever look back longingly on your childhood dreams, it's good to ask yourself some questions:

1. **Is that dream still possible? What would it look like if I pursued it now?** People don't all live their lives in the same order, and sometimes it isn't too late to do something you dreamed of when you were younger. Plenty of people achieve their dreams later in life. Sometimes, however, it is too late, and accepting that is part of moving on.

2. If it is still possible, is it *really* still what I dream of? Our experiences change us and, while we may regret giving up on something we wanted when we were younger, it may not really be what we want now, after all.

Sometimes we may decide it's right to let go of something we once sincerely hoped for and leave it in the past: either we don't want it any more, or we realize it's never going to happen. Perhaps the perfect marriage turned out not to be, or an injury destroyed your hopes of being a professional athlete, or maybe you spent years pursuing a career that involved travel and you've realized you really want to settle down in one place. When we realize it's time to move on from something we once pursued with all our might, it's important that we acknowledge how that makes us feel. When we hope for something, we make it real, if only in our minds. When it doesn't materialize, we feel a sense of loss. If you're grieving for something you once hoped for, take time to do that. Just because it never materialized, it doesn't make the grief any less real.

Whether you want the same thing out of life that you've always wanted, or whether it's time to dream a new dream, working out your values and priorities is likely to translate into a hope or an ambition – to be able to buy your own house, achieve some kind of career success, write a novel or simply have a holiday or a quiet, drama-free life. No dream is too big, too small or too silly. Spend some time thinking about what you want.

TO DO

Spend some time imagining the perfect future: what does it look like? Make a creative representation of that dream, be it a drawing, model, written description or poem: whatever takes your fancy. Put it somewhere you can see it. Whenever you need to, look at it. This can be your happy place.

TO THINK ABOUT

Have a go at filling out the timeline below. Start by thinking about what you want to leave behind, the things that have held you back. From today, there is a fork in the timeline: imagine the future you want and the one you don't want. Nearest to today, write what you want and don't want for the rest of this week/month and, as the timeline extends outward, you can jot down what you want and don't want in the more distant future. You can be as detailed as you like on here; maybe it's a general feeling, or maybe you have specific, detailed plans – write whatever works for you. Knowing the path you don't want to take is just as useful as knowing the path you do want to take, as it can help you say "No" to potential pitfalls.

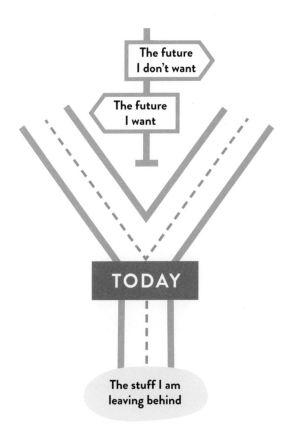

Step 24

To Do

> Without vision the people will perish, and without courage and inspiration, dreams will die.
>
> ROSA PARKS

In this chapter, we have considered what is important to us. Perhaps you now have a clear vision and goal for your future, or perhaps you've got an inkling of an idea.

You may not have an exact plan for what you want the future to look like, but you might know how you want it to feel. You might not know exactly what you want to be doing with your life, but you might know exactly the sort of person you want to be while you're doing it.

That's okay. We don't all have to have a detailed five-year plan; sometimes the journey is as important as the destination. What's important is to understand what success looks like to you and to make sure the things you do match up with that.

If we've been told what success looks like and we've failed to achieve it, or don't even want it, we might feel like we're unsuccessful. However, we all have the right to define success on our own terms.

For example, if you've grown up believing success means getting married and having a nice husband and well-behaved children, but you have ended up divorced and your children are pushing your boundaries, you might feel like "a loser". But it's worth remembering that you aren't necessarily in control of those things, which makes them a poor measure of success. It's also worth asking whether simply "finding a husband and having children" is the most important priority in your life; what about you and what *you* do?

We shouldn't measure our success by other people's behaviour toward us or who we happen to have met because that isn't something we have control over.

Or perhaps you've always believed that success is about wealth: if you have a nice car or house, you're successful; if you're a CEO by 30, you're successful; if you marry a rich man, you're successful. But money isn't everything. Perhaps success looks like happiness rather than stuff, and maybe the sacrifices you would have to make to get the stuff aren't worth it to you? Maybe they would compromise your values?

Write below what success means to you.

Now consider that picture of success and ask yourself the following questions about it:

1. Could I achieve this without compromising my values?

2. When I consider what sort of person I want to be, is that the kind of person who would achieve this kind of success?

3. Is this success reliant on me, or on others?

4. How would I feel if I achieved this?

5. Am I able to achieve this?

If you're finding it hard to work out what success looks like for you, think about what it would feel like. Now try to imagine what would have to be happening in your life for you to feel like that.

To Think About

Hopefully you've had a chance to think about what's most important to you and what you want to be known for. You should also have an idea from the last chapter about the strengths you want to develop. See if you can draw up a plan of these things by completing the sentences below:

My most important value is:

_____

_____

The thing that matters most to me is:

_____

_____

The thing I want to be known for is:

_____

_____

The skill or personality trait I want to develop is:

_____

_____

In the next 12 months, I want to:

_____

_____

In five years' time, I would like to:

_____

_____

TO DO

If you've managed to complete those sentences, then you have an idea of where you're headed. Well done! Now, go back to your To Do list that you wrote in Step 21.

Do the things you do match up with who you want to be?

Will the things you do help or hinder you to grow the way you want to?

If there are things on your list that are hindering your growth, or simply wasting your time, is there a way you can stop doing these things?

Is there anything you want to add or take away from your To Do list?

Step 25

You Are More Than What You Do

> You are valuable because you exist. Not because of what you do or what you have done, but simply because you are.
>
> MAX LUCADO

I once went to listen to Professor Brian Cox talking about time and space. First he explained how tiny our planet is in comparison to all of space. He talked about how, even though there are around 700 quintillion (yes, that is a real number and no, I cannot even imagine how massive it is) planets, there is a high probability that Earth is the only one capable of supporting life. Any life is miraculous and fragile; other planets can't even sustain single-cell organisms, yet you are highly complex, intelligent life.

He then explained that in comparison to how long the universe has existed, the Earth has been in existence for merely the blink of an eye. In comparison to how long the Earth has existed, humanity is young: the dinosaurs ruled the Earth for 135 million years before humanity even existed.

Humanity is both rare and brief. That makes us precious. Of the 100 billion humans who have ever existed, you are the only you. Or, as Professor Cox puts it:

> Look at any randomly selected piece of your world. Encoded deep in the biology of every cell in every blade of grass, in every insect's wing, in every bacterium cell, is the history of the third planet from the Sun in a Solar System making its way

lethargically around a galaxy called the Milky Way. Its shape, form, function, colour, smell, taste, molecular structure, arrangement of atoms, sequence of bases and possibilities for the future are all absolutely unique. There is nowhere else in the observable Universe where you will see precisely that little clump of emergent, living complexity. It is wonderful.

BRIAN COX, *WONDERS OF LIFE: EXPLORING THE MOST EXTRAORDINARY PHENOMENON IN THE UNIVERSE*[18]

Did you get that? In the vastness of the entire universe, you are unique and you are wonderful.

We've spent time considering the importance of what we do. Our existence is brief, so it's good to make the most of it. If we take control and act intentionally, we get to decide who we become, and in that sense, we are what we do.

Yet we are more than what we do, we are more than what we have experienced and we are more than the sum of our genetics. We are each unique, precious and wonderful, no matter what we have done or what has been done to us, no matter what the circumstances of our lives are.

When we spend time living purposefully, it's easy to place our value in what we do. Dream your dreams, set your goals, but always remember: whether you reach your goals or not, you are amazing just for being. What you do makes absolutely no difference to your value. If you fail, you're still amazing. You're still valuable. You don't need to do in order to have worth, you just need to be. If something happens beyond your control to stop you doing the things you planned, that's okay. You can take time out, time spent just being you is never wasted.

[18] Learn more in Brian Cox's *Wonders of Life: Exploring the Most Extraordinary Phenomenon in the Universe* (HarperCollins, 2013).

TO THINK ABOUT

What have you been doing with your time recently? Are you happy with that? Have you been doing too much, too little or just enough? Are you resting? Do you value yourself for who you are or for what you achieve?

_____

_____

_____

_____

_____

_____

_____

_____

_____

_____

_____

_____

_____

_____

To Do

Try a mindfulness meditation. You can find them online, or you can have a go at the chocolate meditation here:

Chocolate meditation

1. Grab yourself a few small pieces of chocolate – any kind of chocolate is fine.

2. Find a comfortable position to sit in, take some deep breaths and relax your body, focusing on relaxing your muscles.

3. Before taking a tiny nibble of the chocolate, take a good look at how delicious it appears. Smell the chocolate and really enjoy its sweet aroma. Finally, take a small bite of the chocolate, then let it melt in your mouth. Continue to breathe deeply and concentrate on the taste of the chocolate.

4. As you swallow the chocolate, focus on the sensations this causes: notice how empty your mouth feels. As you take a second bite of the chocolate, notice how it feels in your hand as you raise your arm to your mouth. Continue to focus on the sensations you are feeling in the present moment.

5. If your mind wanders during your chocolate meditation, gently bring yourself back to the chocolate. The idea is to stay in the present moment as much as you possibly can.

6. When you've finished, you can revisit these feelings throughout your day to feel more relaxed.

Chapter Six

TAKING CARE OF ME

Step 26

It Matters Because You Matter

> Taking care of yourself doesn't mean "me first", it means "me too".
>
> L. R. KNOST

A story...

Once upon a time, there was a poor farmer who only had a small vegetable patch. The farmer worked hard growing and selling vegetables until she saved up enough to buy a goose. When the farmer took her goose home, she was astonished to find that each day it laid an egg made of pure gold. Before long, the farmer was rich. But as the farmer became rich, she also became greedy: she began to demand the goose lay more golden eggs. She beat the goose and told it that it would not be fed until it laid two eggs a day. For the first two weeks, the farmer rubbed her hands in glee as the goose laid more and more eggs each day. But the goose became exhausted: it grew thin and its feathers started to fall out, but still the farmer demanded more eggs. Until one day, the farmer went out to the goose and found it dead. She never had a golden egg again.[19]

Had the farmer taken care of the goose, provided good food and plenty of rest, the goose would have lived a long life, laying even better golden eggs. In the long run, it would have been more profitable.

Sometimes we treat ourselves like the golden goose. We take care of all the other people in our lives: our children, our friends, our families. We run around keeping ourselves busy, seeing rest and recuperation as self-indulgence or selfishness, and we keep churning out the golden eggs while neglecting ourselves – the golden goose.

Previously we considered challenging ourselves to change our environment or do different things. I've suggested doing unfamiliar activities, things that may be contrary to your nature, and pushing yourself outside your comfort zone. All that stuff is hard work. It's physically and emotionally tiring. If you're doing this, then you also need to rest and recharge your batteries.

Remember your To Do list? We talked about prioritizing the things that will help you grow and achieve your goals. Is rest and self-care on there? It should be. If you want to grow physically, mentally and emotionally, rest is vital.

Just as our personalities and experiences are all unique, so is the way we rest, recuperate and find joy. Ultimately, it starts with believing you have the right to put yourself first from time to time and realizing that sometimes it's good to just...

Stop.

[19] This story has been inspired by one of Aesop's fables – the goose that laid the golden eggs. Read more in *Aesop's Fables*, a new translation by V. S. Vernon Jones (London: W. Heinemann, 1912).

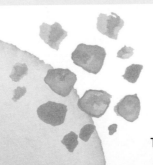

TO THINK ABOUT

Do you believe you have the right to put yourself first?

Do you believe you are important and worthy of kindness?

Do you believe it's okay to spend time doing absolutely nothing?

Do you allow yourself to do that?

To Do

Remember the happy little monster we discussed in Step 10? Go back and look at the monster you created. Would you draw it the same way now? Has it become friendlier, or angrier? Have you been feeding your monster a diet of kindness?

What was your positive affirmation? Do you now believe this? Is it time to change your positive affirmation for something even more positive, or something else you need to work on?

Is there any negativity you've dealt with and removed from your life since you created your little monster? If so, can you chuck it in the Fuck-It Bucket? Or perhaps you can chuck the notion of being unkind to yourself – of denying yourself rest – in the Fuck-It Bucket?

Step 27

Be Your Own Best Friend

> I hope... that you will, when you need to be, be wise,
> and that you will always be kind.
>
> NEIL GAIMAN

What do you look for in a friend? Write on the picture opposite what the perfect best friend or companion would be like. How would they treat you?

Now have a read about my best friend:

My best friend reminds me regularly that I'm valuable, funny and clever. When she goes to the supermarket, she thinks about me and picks me up little treats, such as a pack of biscuits or a cake. In the mornings, my best friend makes me a cup of tea and reminds me of the importance of a good breakfast; she tells me to eat healthily, but she also makes sure I don't beat myself up when I get a takeaway because I can't be bothered to cook. My best friend laughs at my bad jokes and tells me I'm hilarious. When I make mistakes, she reminds me that I have the right not to be perfect: she won't allow me to feel shame. When I get home from a long day, she tells me it's okay to put my feet up and rest; she doesn't care if I take my bra off, and she lets me have a cry and a moan if I need to. She's great company; we go to the cinema together, sometimes we pop into a nice coffee shop and treat ourselves to cake or go for a drive in my camper van, or sometimes we simply sit quietly with a brew and a book.

Sounds great, doesn't she? Do you know who my best friend is?

It's me!

What did you decide you would want from a friend?

Do you do those things for yourself, or just for others? Kindness is wonderful and we should all be kind at every given opportunity, but kindness isn't just for other people – it's for ourselves, too. We all deserve kindness, and we're equally as deserving of our own kindness as our friends are.

So, next time you're chastising yourself, think, "Would I talk to my best friend like this?" When you see that bunch of pretty daffodils in the supermarket, consider: would you buy them for your friend? In that case, grab a bunch for yourself as well! If you want someone fun to hang out with, go have fun enjoying your own company: it may seem scary walking into a coffee shop or the cinema on your own, but once you've mastered it, it's empowering.

Be your own best friend.

Maybe you think you need to wait for your Prince Charming to arrive to provide you with your "Happily Ever After", but why sit around waiting for some chance encounter, or waiting for fortune to smile on you? You don't need Prince Charming or anyone else to take care of you: you hold the keys to your own happiness, so don't put them in someone else's pocket.

Of course, that's not to say that relationships with others aren't necessary or fulfilling. This is why it's important to be kind to others, too, but enjoying the company of others is different to needing it for your own well-being and happiness. If you leave the responsibility of making you feel happy to others, you're effectively just leaving it to chance.

TO THINK ABOUT

Revisit the circles of control and circles of concern that we looked at in Step 20. Where would you put your need to feel loved or your need for happiness? Are they within your circle of concern, or your circle of control? What about other people's happiness? Where would you put that?

To Do

Think of a random act of kindness that you can do for someone you care about this week. Then do it for yourself as well. How did these acts of kindness make you feel?

_____

_____

_____

_____

_____

_____

_____

_____

_____

_____

_____

_____

Step 28

My Happy Place

> Happiness is the best makeup.
>
> DREW BARRYMORE

A few years ago, professional organizer Marie Kondo[20] went viral with her notion that you should only keep items around you that "spark joy". I'm not too sure I agree with that: my washing machine doesn't particularly "spark joy", but it's probably best that I don't throw it away. However, I do love the notion that there are things, people, places and activities that can make you feel joyful in an instant. Can you imagine that "Ahhh" feeling? For me, it's the feeling I get when I take the first sip of tea in the morning, or when I step outside my front door on a sunny spring weekend and all my tulips have opened. Fill in the mind map below with things that spark joy in you.

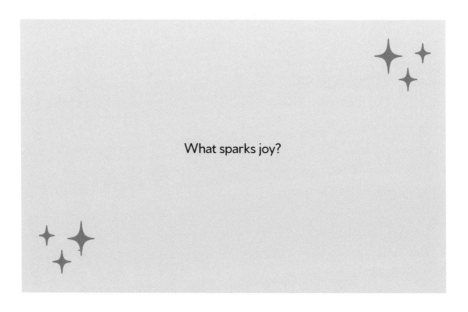

What sparks joy?

When we think about "self-care", we may think about long soaks in the bath and pamper nights, but that's not for everyone. Our different personality traits mean that different things make us feel happy or relaxed, we all have different ways of recharging. That's okay. Do what makes you happy.

Tick the statements below that apply to you, to help you think about the best ways you can rest and recharge:

- [ ] I am happier enjoying my own company.
- [ ] I prefer to be with friends/ family than on my own.
- [ ] I like quiet time.
- [ ] I prefer to be active.
- [ ] I'm easily bored.
- [ ] I love learning new things.

- [ ] I prefer to not have to think too deeply when I'm chilling out.
- [ ] I could sit around for an hour doing nothing.
- [ ] My happiness is easily affected by the behaviour of others.
- [ ] My happiness is rooted in how I feel about myself.

It's also good to have a place you can go where you feel calm and can de-stress and recharge. Maybe you're unable to create a sanctuary right now. That's okay: you can create a fantasy happy place where you can go in your mind any time. Mine is a log cabin in a silent wood, with a squishy armchair and a log fire. Perhaps yours is a tent at a festival, or a beach in the Caribbean, or perhaps it's the future dream you imagined for yourself in the last chapter.

Create this place in your mind, sparing no details: what does it look like? Smell like? Is it warm? Cold? What are you sitting or lying on? How does it feel underneath you? Are you indoors? Outdoors? What can you hear? Whenever you need to relax, go to this place in your mind.

[20] To learn more about Marie Kondo, watch her show on Netflix, or read *Spark Joy: An Illustrated Master Class on the Art of Organizing and Tidying Up* by Marie Kondo (Ten Speed Press, 2016).

To Do

Draw your happy place...

See if you can practise visiting your happy place every day this week. You can do it any time: it only takes five minutes. Just close your eyes, slow your breathing and then go through each of your five senses as you imagine yourself there: what does it look, sound, smell, feel and taste like (perhaps you can taste the salt in the sea air, or the smoke from your campfire)? When you open your eyes, do you feel more relaxed?

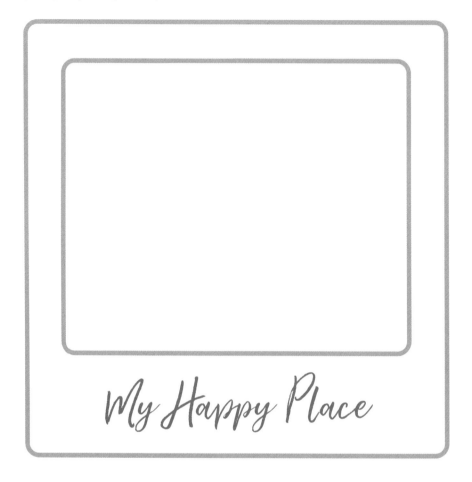

My Happy Place

TO THINK ABOUT

It's good to schedule dedicated time for yourself, but sometimes you may not be able to do this. It may be that things are getting on top of you right in the middle of a hectic day. How can you find breathing space in your day? What two- to five-minute things can you do to re-centre yourself in the middle of a day?

Step 29

Planning Self-Care

> I have met myself and I am going to care for her fiercely.
>
> GLENNON DOYLE

Rest and relaxation are important aspects of self-care, but there's more to it than that. It's about making sure our needs are met – physically, mentally, emotionally, spiritually, financially and more. For example, think about how we care for children: of course, we help them learn to relax, calm them down when they're stressed and show them kindness. But we also make sure they're eating healthily, cleaning their teeth and doing their homework. We give them pocket money to teach them to manage their finances; we arrange playdates to help them form relationships; we teach them right from wrong and put boundaries in place. This is what self-care is about for us, too. It's not just about taking "me time" occasionally – it's about making sure every aspect of our lives is as healthy as it possibly can be.

Self-care is something that should be an ongoing part of each and every day. It doesn't have to always be long walks or pamper nights; sometimes a five-minute recharge is enough. Sometimes, in the midst of chaos, it's enough to excuse yourself to the toilet, sit down, close your eyes, breathe and go to your happy place, before heading back into the fray. Five-minute recharges include that mid-morning brew and biscuit; the kind word you speak to yourself on the way to a meeting; the time it takes to apply hand cream after washing your hands; or replying to a text from a friend.

In fact, you may not even have to stop to recharge. Sometimes, a change really is as good as a rest. If I've had a very "people-y" morning, I may spend my afternoon quietly doing some admin: I'm still working, but I'm recharging my batteries by switching my activity.

This is especially helpful if the activity you've been doing is outside your natural comfort zone. As an extrovert, if I spend a day alone working on quiet tasks, I can feel more exhausted than if I've spent a day running between meetings. In this instance, I wouldn't recharge by having a quiet evening in, I'd recharge by socializing.

Similarly, an introvert may have to recharge after socializing. If you are an introvert, you may need to set boundaries by saying "No" to some social engagements if you find them hard: that's self-care. It may be you know you're going to be doing lots of activities that you find exhausting, so it's important that day to build in some moments when you can recharge. Knowing your limits, and understanding what you find tiring and what you find revitalizing, is key to a healthy self-care plan.

All the things you have discovered about yourself are vital to your self-care plan: what you know about your strengths and weaknesses; your likes and dislikes; what you find comfortable and what you don't; where you're heading; and how you're spending your time will inform you about the sort of things you need to be doing to recharge in order to stay healthy and happy.

To Think About

Go back and look at the tree you drew in Step 4. Your tree was about how you want to grow and what you want your life to look like. Are you still happy with this? If you want to, you can make changes to your tree now.

Now look at your To Do list from Step 21. If you complete the things on your To Do list, will your tree grow how you want it to? If not, make some changes to your To Do list: add anything you need to and remove anything you don't need to be doing. Do you need to throw anything in the Fuck-It Bucket?

To Do

Below is an example of a self-care plan, explaining what kind of things to consider in each area of your life. Remember, not every act of self-care needs to be time-consuming – sometimes it's as simple as ensuring your environment is a calm and nurturing place you want to spend time in. On the following page is a blank copy of a self-care plan. Have a go at making one for yourself. Then commit to taking care of yourself in these ways.

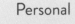

Physical

Sleep
Heathy food
Rest
Exercise
Physical release

Personal

Knowing yourself
Being true to your values
Hobbies
Personal identity

Financial

Budgeting
Saving
Treats
Paying bills

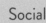

Spiritual

Time alone
Time in nature
Connection
Prayer or meditation
Journalling
Reading

Emotional

Managing stress
Emotional awareness
Compassion
Kindness
Building resilience

Space

Safety
Security
Stability
Warmth
Ventilation
Clean/tidy

Social

Boundaries
Support systems
Positive relationships
Communication
Asking for help
Time together

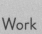

Work

Time management
Boundaries
Positive environment
Breaks
Development

Self-Care Plan

Physical

_____
_____
_____
_____
_____
_____

Personal

_____
_____
_____
_____
_____

Financial

_____
_____
_____
_____
_____

Spiritual

_____
_____
_____
_____

Emotional

_____
_____
_____
_____

Space

_____
_____
_____
_____
_____

Work

_____
_____
_____
_____

Social

_____
_____
_____
_____
_____

Step 30

What Now?

> You're off to great places! Today is your day!
> Your mountain is waiting, So... get on your way.
>
> **DR SEUSS**

We've reached the end of our journey together. How's it been?

We've thought about our natural traits and our experiences, and how they contribute to make us the person we are. We've looked at how the things we do affect how we grow and who we become. We've considered how we can build our strengths and reinvent our weaknesses as a force for good, and how we can take control of our superpowers to make a difference in our corner of the world. We've chosen to be kind to ourselves and be our own best friend. We've chucked stuff in the Fuck-It Bucket, and hopefully got rid of guilt, shame and unkindness toward ourselves; and we've considered how we can take charge of our journey and personal growth. We hold the keys to our own happiness and our own future, and from now on, we're taking charge of writing our own story. Hopefully, you've got to know yourself a bit better – and learned to like yourself a bit more, too. Perhaps you've got a lovely pet monster now who speaks kindly to you?

On reflection

I've tried to include lots of different exercises for reflection in this book – journalling, drawing, creating art, reading, thinking and meditation. Not all of these will have worked for you. Maybe none of them have, or maybe there's been something you've really enjoyed doing, which you can now build into your schedule moving forward. Make sure you keep making time for you – time to reflect on how it's going, and to do the things that work for you and get rid of the things that don't.

TO THINK ABOUT

Here are a few questions to consider about your journey so far:

What stands out to you most about what you've got from your journey?

_____

_____

_____

_____

_____

What will you do differently now?

_____

_____

_____

_____

_____

What do you like most about yourself?

_____

_____

_____

_____

_____

To Do – Fuck It!

Now would be a great opportunity to get rid of the contents of your Fuck-It Bucket! I hope you've found some nonsense you don't need that you're ready to let go of. Maybe you've thrown away baggage foisted on you by others. Maybe you've thought about stereotypes you hold about part of your identity and have said, "Fuck it – I can be whoever I want to be." Or maybe you've thrown away some untrue thoughts you've had about yourself. I hope you've managed to remove some of the dead weights that may be holding you down so you can spread your wings and enjoy your freedom. Now, what are you going to do with all those bits of paper in your Fuck-It Bucket? If you have access to a shredder, you could shred them, or if you can get outside and do so safely, you could burn them. Or maybe you'll just tear them up yourself. Destroying the symbols of the things that have kept us trapped and have stopped us being everything we are can be truly cathartic and empowering. Enjoy it!

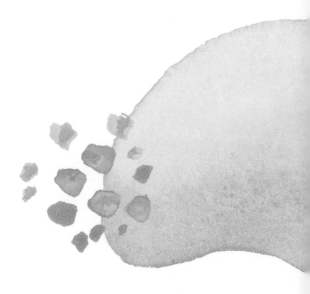

SO, WHAT ARE YOUR NEXT STEPS?

I can't answer that – only you can. You have your tree, you know how you want to grow, and you have your To Do list – all that's left is for you to do it. But remember, whatever you do, do it with kindness. Kindness to others and kindness to yourself. You determine what success looks like to you, not others, and whether you achieve your dreams or not, you're no less valuable, worthy and precious. Always hold on to that. And don't forget to rest and, sometimes, to simply stop and reflect.

I hope you've enjoyed this journal and that it's proved positive and helpful. Most of all, I hope that whatever you do next, you do it with a little bit of love for who you are. You're amazing.

Go confidently in the direction of your dreams. Live the life you have imagined.

HENRY DAVID THOREAU

ABOUT THE AUTHOR

Sally Hope is a recovery coach with a specialism in supporting women who have experienced domestic abuse. Sally uses her personal experience of trauma recovery, alongside her professional knowledge and her gentle, down-to-earth humour, to empower women to live lives full of joy and hope. She is passionate about humanity, personal growth, faith, spirituality, laughter, campervanning with her children and LEGO.

You can connect with Sally on Facebook where she posts uplifting and thought-provoking content: www.facebook.com/sallyhopealwayshopeful

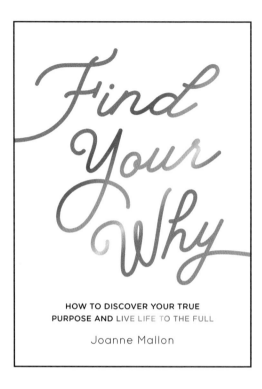

HOW TO DISCOVER YOUR TRUE
PURPOSE AND LIVE LIFE TO THE FULL

Joanne Mallon

FIND YOUR WHY

How to Discover Your True Purpose and Live Life to the Full

Joanne Mallon

Paperback

978-1-78783-998-4

Knowing your purpose, or your "why", has the power to transform your life – and this book will help you to discover yours. From reflecting on your past to visualizing your future, the tips and advice in these pages will guide you towards your true calling, and a deeper sense of contentment and happiness.

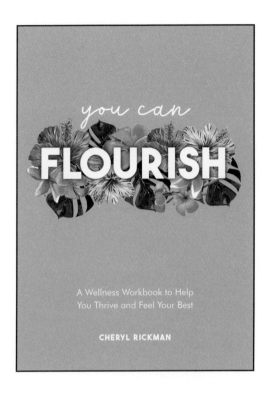

YOU CAN FLOURISH

A Wellness Workbook to Help You Thrive and Feel Your Best

Cheryl Rickman

Paperback

978-1-80007-681-5

Feeling better isn't always about feeling good. It's about feeling it all – happiness, sadness and everything in between. In *You Can Flourish*, Positive Psychology Practitioner Cheryl Rickman takes you step by step through simple exercises to help you better experience both the positive and negative in life, so you can thrive and grow.

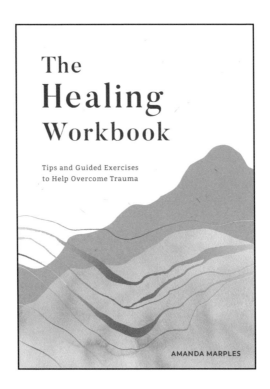

THE HEALING WORKBOOK

Tips and Guided Exercises to Help Overcome Trauma

Amanda Marples

Paperback

978-1-80007-768-3

Begin your healing journey with this step-by-step workbook to help you understand and deal with trauma. Including practical advice, effective tips and guided exercises based on trusted CBT techniques it will help you to process the past and find your way back to yourself, your values, and a life where you can flourish and thrive.

IMAGE CREDITS

Have you enjoyed this book?

If so, why not write a review on your favourite website?

If you're interested in finding out more about our books, find us on Facebook at **Summersdale Publishers**, on Twitter at **@Summersdale** and on Instagram and TikTok at **@summersdalebooks** and get in touch. We'd love to hear from you!

Thanks very much for buying this Summersdale book.

www.summersdale.com